DEAD CENTER

DEAD
CENTER

BEHIND THE SCENES AT THE WORLD'S LARGEST MEDICAL EXAMINER'S OFFICE

SHIYA RIBOWSKY

AND TOM SHACHTMAN

REGAN

An Imprint of HarperCollinsPublishers

To preserve their anonymity, we have changed the names of some individuals and modified identifying features, including physical descriptions and occupations of other individuals. In some cases, composite characters have been created or timelines have been compressed, to further preserve privacy and to maintain narrative flow. The goal in all cases was to protect people's privacy without damaging the integrity of the story.

HarperCollins books may be purchased for educational, business, or sales promotional use. For information please write: Special Markets Department, HarperCollins Publishers Inc., 10 East 53rd Street, New York, NY 10022.

FIRST EDITION

Designed by Publications Development Company of Texas

Library of Congress Cataloging-in-Publication Data has been applied for.

ISBN 10: 0-06-111624-6

ISBN 13: 978-0-06-111624-7

06 07 08 09 10 PDC/RRD 10 9 8 7 6 5 4 3 2 1

Dead-ication

To my dear wife Jennifer, who astonishingly chose me and whose love gives me the courage to reach higher.

To Chava, Reena, Eli, and Jake, I love you.
May your lives be full of delightful choices.

To Rock Positano and to R.A.H.

"Show me the manner in which a nation cares for its dead, and I will measure with mathematical exactness, the tender mercies of its people, their loyalty to high ideals, and their regard for the laws of the land."

—William Ewart Gladstone, 1809–1898

INTRODUCTION

THE MORNING OF September 11, 2001, was sunny and crystal clear—the kind of day that is too rare in New York City—with perfect temperature and no humidity. I arrived as usual at my office at 8:00 A.M., after the six-block walk from my apartment, coffee and muffin in hand. It was such a beautiful day that I decided to have my breakfast outside, sitting on the edge of a granite flowerbed, while I awaited my first visitor of the morning.

I looked up at the building where I worked, the Office of the Chief Medical Examiner of New York (OCME). After working there for eleven years, I still thought of it affectionately as the ugliest building in Manhattan: a misshapen turquoise rectangle on the corner of Thirtieth Street and First Avenue, adjacent to New York University Hospital. A testament to 1950s municipal-pile architecture, the building was an amusing embarrassment to all who worked within.

My visitor was Dr. Steve Schwartz, registrar and assistant commissioner of New York City's vital statistics office (at the Department of Health), the repository of every birth and death certificate issued in the city. By 8:30 A.M., we were in a meeting inside. My title at OCME was director of identifications, and we had gathered that morning to discuss

New York City's Electronic Death Registration System (EDRS), a system designed to allow OCME and hospitals to file death certificates with the health department via the Internet. This costly project had been started and delayed many times; now we were trying to determine how to get it back on track.

Such a system would be very useful, one of us pointed out early in the meeting, in the case of a mass fatality.

Shortly before 9:00 A.M., our meeting was interrupted by Nick Fusco, OCME's facilities manager, who stuck his head in the office and told us that a plane had hit the World Trade Center (WTC). And that I might want to get myself to the conference room, which had the only television set on the premises.

As I hurried through the corridors, my mind flashed back to an incident from the previous weekend. I'd noticed a small plane, circling illegally at very low altitude over Manhattan's East Side, towing a banner protesting something having to do with the United Nations and human rights. *Uh-oh*, I thought, *that idiot's back again, and his Piper Cub, or whatever it was, has hit one of the towers.*

In the conference room, I joined a group of colleagues huddled grimly around the television set. One glance at the televised image of the tower burning, and I threw out my Piper Cub theory. No small plane could have caused that amount of damage: the tower looked as though it had been nuked.

I was shocked. But immediately, almost involuntarily, my mind flooded with professional questions. How many people had died? How many were injured? How would we identify the victims? How would we transport the bodies to the office for processing? Where would we handle the processing?

Then the next plane hit, and I felt something more: fear. The first plane might have been an accident, but the second left no room for misunderstanding. This was an attack—right here, on my city, my country. On an intellectual level, I must have understood what was going on, but it took hours for me to *believe* that the event unfolding before my eyes was actually happening.

During the brief period when just the first tower was ablaze, before the second plane hit, I had felt awful about the victims, but I had remained calm. Now I was scared: fearful for my loved ones, my country, my city, and perhaps even for myself.

Reports began to come in about more attacks—that additional planes were inbound, that a truck had just detonated on the George Washington Bridge. Thankfully, those and similar reports proved to be false, but as the terrible day wore on, we learned that a third plane had attacked the Pentagon and that a fourth hijacked plane had crashed in Pennsylvania.

My thoughts coursed onward in parallel tracks, one worried for the safety and well-being of my loved ones, for those in the towers, and for my country; the other engaged with professional concerns. I also became aware that I was reacting to the strain in other ways. For one thing, I noticed a metallic taste in my mouth; I came to think of it as the nickel taste, and it would stay with me for weeks, a physical manifestation of my emotional stress.

Within the first half-hour of the tragedy, the OCME began to deploy its initial response. Dr. Charles Hirsch, chief medical examiner (CME), and a group of other staff members had gathered in front of the building, preparing to head downtown. The towers had not yet fallen; none of us even suspected that they might collapse. The plan was for the "away" team to reconnoiter at the site and then contact us with instructions on what we were facing and how to prepare. They would also locate and secure appropriate locations for temporary field morgues.

I wanted to go downtown with the chief, and at first I was disappointed when he told me to stay behind at the office. But somebody had to remain at headquarters to prepare for the task ahead. Whatever bodies were recovered at the site would have to be processed and identified, and as director of identifications for the office and senior medicolegal investigator (MLI) for Manhattan, it fell to me to start organizing our efforts.

In a sense, too, I was relieved. I wasn't sure there would be much for our agency to do at the site, whereas the job of preparing the main office for the tasks to come was bound to be challenging. After all, I reasoned, it would be hours before the fires were put out, and more hours before the injured were attended to. Only then would full attention be paid to the dead. I went back into the building to look for another MLI to go with Dr. Hirsch. Three of my colleagues were in the lobby. One of them, Dianne Crisci, half-jokingly pleaded, "Hey, pick me, pick me!"

"You want it, you got it," I said, and walked her outside to join Dr. Hirsch, anthropologist Amy Mundorff, and six other staff members, all equipped with Nextel phones and two-way radios. Going downtown in several vehicles, they soon reached what the world would shortly come to know as Ground Zero.

From their initial reports, it could as easily have been labeled Hell on Earth.

At the office, we listened over phones and radios to our seasoned coworkers crying as they watched people jump from the burning towers.

"My God, my God this is awful—the noise the bodies make when they hit!"

"We're walking over body parts here, Shiya. Bodies everywhere. You'd better start getting some refrigerated trucks—we're not gonna have enough room for all these bodies."

Then the South Tower fell, and we immediately lost contact with Dr. Hirsch and his team as the antenna that routed much of the city's mobile phone traffic fell with the building. Busy on my end in the communications unit, I missed the fall of the tower. But shouts of dismay summoned me back to the conference room, in time to watch as the North Tower followed at 10:29 A.M. The conference room was full but hushed, save for the saddened voices of the television commentators, and a colleague's quiet sobbing. After the second tower fell, we stood watching the television and mourning for a few moments more; then, one by one, we left the room to head back to work.

In that moment, uncertain whether our coworkers were dead or alive, I felt terrible—not just about the tragedy, but about how OCME had reacted. We were not a first-responder agency, but we'd acted as though we were, rushing to the site to deal with a situation without taking the time to assess it properly. Worse yet, we had allowed our agency head to be part of the field team. Now, we were on our own.

Even though we didn't yet know whether we had lost our leader and colleagues, we still had to act—and act immediately. Unfortunately, at that moment many of us had fallen into a kind of shock. Among them was my immediate boss, the agency's chief of staff and director of investigations. Many others were wandering around, looking lost, and awaiting direction.

But when direction wasn't immediately forthcoming, I was unable to sit still. So I set my mind on the first task I could think of: creating a body receiving area and processing system.

Standing nearby was Dave Eibert, commanding officer of the New York Police Department's (NYPD) Missing Persons squad. I had no authority over Dave, or any NYPD officer, but I wasn't thinking about authority. "You, come with me," I said, and we marched off toward the morgue. Later, I couldn't remember barking such an order, but when reminiscing with Dave, he said he didn't give it a second thought. "At that point, I would've followed anyone with a plan," he recalls.

I'm glad he didn't ask me if I had one.

On our way to the morgue, I grabbed two friends, Dr. Mark Flomenbaum, our first deputy chief medical examiner, and Dr. Robert Shaler, head of our DNA lab. We reached the morgue and began to set up a process to examine the remains from the WTC tragedies—a process that would continue, twenty-four hours a day, seven days a week, for almost a year.

As we walked, the outline of a plan was starting to take shape in my head. I had been working as a medicolegal investigator and identification expert since 1989, when Dr. Hirsch had taken over the OCME and began transforming it into the cutting-edge operation it is today. I had not only medical but also forensic and legal training, and before 9/11 my tasks at OCME had routinely called on all of those skills. But far more important, that day and on the days that followed, was something I'd never learned in school—my basic mind-set. By nature I love making order out of chaos.

And it was chaos that confronted us that day—an enormous, overwhelming, and heartbreaking task that would absorb our every waking moment, and many of our nonwaking moments, for the next three years. As a logistical challenge, it was unlike anything we had ever imagined; later I would compare it to building an airplane, in flight, at night, during a storm, with no cockpit light, and only a set of badly translated instructions to guide us.

Late that afternoon, our chief, Dr. Hirsch, made it back to the building. He had almost been killed when the first building came down. Dianne Crisci, the MLI who had begged me to send her to accompany Dr. Hirsch, was standing next to him when the towers collapsed, and she did not make it back to the office that day. Both wounded by a chunk of concrete falling from the upper floors of a tower, Dr. Hirsch and Crisci had been taken to a medical facility in New Jersey. Dr. Hirsch refused treatment for himself, and lingered at the hospital long enough to make sure that Dianne was being properly cared for—her injuries were severe, though she would survive—before bumming a ride with some Port Authority cops back into Manhattan.

Dr. Hirsch's appearance shocked us. He was bruised and battered, with a large laceration on his hand that required suturing. The shock wave that had hit him was so powerful that it had impregnated his clothing with gray dust and pebbles—the residue of what had been reinforced concrete. We insisted that he go next door to New York University Hospital's emergency room. Before he left, he reached into his pocket and pulled out a handful of dust and concrete chips. I spread a paper napkin on his desk, and he emptied the dust onto it. Today that dust is still on his desk in a special container.

A few impressions and recollections from these early days: Pinning on an American flag lapel pin and never taking it off, transferring it from my suit jacket to my suspenders and back, and later proudly wearing a pin of our flag handed to me by former President George H. W. Bush. Being cornered by former President Bill Clinton at the city's Emergency Operations Center along the Hudson River, on Pier 92, eager to talk with Tom Shephardson of Disaster Mortuary Operational Response Team (DMORT) and me about how he had tried and failed to have the CIA kill Osama bin Laden. Having a private conversation with Mayor Giuliani at 2:00 A.M. in a dark corner of the medical examiner's office when he came there to identify the body of a friend. Being so proudly overwhelmed at the quality of work that our office was doing, and of the assistance we were getting, that I thought: *They've killed some of us and brought out the best in the rest of us.*

In those frenzied early days, we all felt grateful to be in a position to help—to do something, anything, to help assuage the pain that the attacks had caused. During the first few weeks after the disaster, when we left the OCME office and saw people applauding the police vehicles we were traveling in, I think we all shared that sense of gratitude. We were all coming together, as New Yorkers and Americans, to help.

I found myself thinking in those days of how often my grandfathers had reminded me and my siblings of how lucky we were to live in the "golden land," where we had security and protection from persecution and where opportunities abounded. Too young to have served in the Vietnam War, and not sure I would have willingly done so, I nevertheless admired those who served our country. I thought of the OCME's effort after 9/11 as similar to a medic's tour of duty in Vietnam, at least when it came to the psychological battering we all took as a result. The relentless arrival of new remains, the onslaught of grief coming from the families—it was difficult to handle such a ceaseless flow of death, even for experienced ME personnel who had spent our careers working with the deceased and the bereaved. Some of us bowed to the stress, retreating from our work to rest and regroup; a few never returned. I kept working, but that doesn't mean I wasn't scarred.

Everyone in New York City, and the surrounding suburbs, seemed to know someone who had perished in the attacks. For a while, I thought I was the exception, but that was only because at first I had so little contact with my usual outside world.

Then, on one of my infrequent trips back to my apartment to change clothes and grab a few hours of sleep, I learned just how out of touch I was. I'd been up for maybe seventy-two hours when a woman whom I vaguely recognized as a neighbor approached me in my apartment building's lobby. "Don't you work for the medical examiner's office?" she asked. I told her I did, but I was tired and irritable, and I was a bit abrupt with her. Sweetly ignoring my tone, she told me that her husband was one of the victims of the attacks and that she needed my help. Mortified by the way I'd spoken, I apologized and told her I hadn't known of her loss. "Of course," she said, "you haven't been home since this happened." A few days later, the news came even closer to home when I learned that a dear friend, Jeffery Weiner, the assistant cantor of my temple, had also been killed.

By day three after the attacks, Dr. Hirsch had formally confirmed me in the position I'd already assumed: director of the identification effort for the WTC victims. I couldn't help feeling that, in some way, it was a job for which I'd been training most of my adult life. Yet, as I ran myself ragged trying to keep up with the pace of the work, burning through mobile-phone batteries, I was also overcome by moments of profound sadness that tempered the adrenaline rush of the work. Still I pushed on, as we all did, rarely giving a thought to the outside world.

In those early weeks, I was unable to leave my post long enough to perform my usual weekend duties as cantor at a temple in Manhattan. But with late September came the holiest of Jewish holidays, Yom Kippur, and I had pledged to the rabbi that I'd make it back to sing the most solemn prayer of all, the *Kol Nidre,* on the eve of the day of atonement.

Suddenly, as I was immersed in work at the Incident Command Center, I realized that sundown was approaching, and with it the start of Yom Kippur. I had only a few minutes to get to the synagogue, about a mile across town. My heart sank; I felt sure there was no way I could make it. But some police officers from Long Island had been working with us, and I asked them if they'd mind taking me. They immediately put me in their car, and off we went. I think I can safely say that I was the only cantor in America who arrived at his synagogue that day in a police cruiser, sirens blaring.

ONE

WHEN PEOPLE ASK what I do for a living, I have two answers. The first, that I work for the medical examiner's (ME) office, usually generates interest on its own, especially in these crime-drama days. The second, that I'm the cantor of a large Manhattan synagogue, is likewise good for a certain amount of conversation, especially among those who remember the cantors of their childhood intoning the *Kol Nidre* during Yom Kippur.

For some reason, though—perhaps because of that old saw about the whole being greater than the sum of its parts—when I tell people about my two jobs, they seem to find the combination a source of decided fascination. Many strangers find it odd, these simultaneous careers in forensics and religious music, and some days it is fairly odd to me. I wonder if there's ever been another medicolegal investigator (MLI) who's worked a double homicide in the morning and conducted synagogue services at dusk. How did a nice Jewish boy from the Orthodox community in Brooklyn end up this way, fussing around with dead people for a living?

The reasons involve history—the Orthodox community's and my own within it.

The early years of the twentieth century saw an enormous influx of Jewish immigrants from Eastern Europe to New York City, a veritable Ashkenazi tidal wave. Many immigrants hit the shores of the "golden land" and quickly merged into the mainstream culture of the melting pot, throwing off the shackles of Old World traditions that now felt too old-fashioned. But quite a few held on to the ancient practices, and the more observant of the immigrants opened kosher food shops and *yeshivot* (Jewish parochial schools), built synagogues and ritual baths, and tried to keep alive—through dress, language, and custom—the culture they had once had in Europe. Doing so wasn't easy, because the general drift of American culture in those years was toward the secular. But their efforts to retain their cultural identity were passionate and won them a place in the urban fabric of the times.

Change in New York City's Ashkenazi community continued at a slow pace during the Depression and World War II. But the two decades after the end of World War II were years of dramatic growth and equally dramatic consolidation of the community. Into the early 1960s, the *Frum* community, as observant Jews call themselves, saw many adherents become more secular and less observant as they were forced to seek jobs outside the community, experience some of the culture of that outside world, and become more interdependent with it. In America, they did not have the insulation from secular influences that they had been used to in Europe—that accorded by the *shtetl*, the insular villages where Jews had lived. In the United States, Jewish sons and daughters could go to universities, to medical and law schools, open businesses, or work in a wide variety of fields, and many did.

My parents, both born in the United States before the end of World War II, were typical Orthodox Jews of their generation. Fully observant of all Jewish law, they raised me, my older sister, and my younger brother in a strictly kosher home in which the highlight of the week was the Sabbath. My father always wore a *yarmulke* or skull cap, and my mother, as a married woman, dutifully covered her head in public. But they had also been secularly educated, and they were fully integrated into modern society without sacrificing their beliefs or practices.

My father George's varied businesses—at one time or another he was the proprietor of a carpet store, a commercial bakery, a wholesale food distributor, and a check-cashing store—certainly brought him in touch with the outside world. My mother Helene, who has a PhD degree, had a thriving private practice in special education and had been a university professor; she, too, was clearly comfortable in the wider world.

As the 1960s wore on, there was a perceptible shift within the Frum community in a different direction—away from the modern world. Partially in reaction to its members' increasing secularism, and partially because the Frum community was now numerous and wealthy enough to afford the move back toward its roots, it began to do so. The Orthodox became more orthodox, more observant of the myriad laws governing daily existence and ritual, more conservative, and more insular. Another pressure pushing this return to fundamentalism was the psychological makeup of a community whose members considered themselves to be collective Holocaust survivors. By 1965, when I was born, the community had already launched a drive to re-create, in the New York Orthodox community, the Frum lifestyle of pre–World War II Eastern Europe.

My childhood was filled with stories of the wonderful *Yiddishe* life of the old country, told on countless occasions during my early school years by the rabbis of our religious schools and neighborhood synagogues. It was our obligation, they told us, to cling ever more tightly to the ways of our ancestors now that Hitler had killed six million of our relatives but failed to eradicate Jews as a people. For us to survive and to be more religious as a community and as individuals would signify the ultimate defeat of the terrible hatred that the Third Reich had embodied.

This drive to fundamentalism meant that people born into the Frum community in the 1960s and afterward were faced with a choice. They had to decide which side of the line they would be on: the side of the Hebrew/Yiddish/Frum culture, or the other, secular side that we called the *Goyishe* culture. If members wanted to be secular—or didn't want to be quite as observant as others in the community—they left the culture behind, either drifting away slowly or making a decisive break. In either instance, the community often cemented such choices in place behind the former member: when you left, you left everyone you grew up with. Indeed, families sometimes even chose to sever close relations with kin who abandoned the Frum for the outside world.

The twenty years between my parents' generation and mine saw tremendous changes in how orthodoxy was practiced—right down to the way the Frum dressed or named their children. In the 1940s, my grandparents had wanted their children to fit in. They chose to adopt English-sounding names for my parents, which helped them not to stand out—a desirable thing to the Holocaust generation, for whom standing out was a terrifying prospect. Twenty years later, though, the Jewish community was beginning to feel safe and at home in America; that's why my parents felt comfortable naming me Shiya, and giving my brother a name with one of those "ch" syllables that makes it difficult to pronounce. By the time we were born, my parents' common English names were no longer considered appropriate for a Frum child; I would have been mercilessly teased in yeshiva (Jewish parochial school) with a moniker like George.

Despite the fact that my parents had grown up in a relatively re-laxed Orthodox community, by the time that I arrived, they had moved along with the swing to the right and were solidly in the Frum culture. This made sense for our family, whose roots were deep in the Orthodox Jewish community and culture. Growing up I heard as much Yiddish as English, and it was impressed on me that learned rabbinical scholars abounded in our family tree as far back as we could follow it. Such scholars are also well represented in the family's current generations. Cantors also abound in the family; in fact, you can't throw a prayer book at a family reunion without hitting one (or at least someone who thinks he is a cantor).

For grade school, I attended a yeshiva in Brooklyn, one that I have to characterize in retrospect as a very conservative academy—conser-vative in both the religious and the political senses. It was a parochial school that relied heavily on the traditional and religious aspects of Jewish culture, with instruction in secular subjects being an after-thought at best. The school's administration was aware of the state's minimum guidelines and met them—barely. Most graduates of this yeshiva would not go on to secular education at any level; a few would continue their religious studies on through adulthood, and during the rest of their lives would do nothing else but study the Talmud, the compendium of Jewish law and tradition begun two thousand years ago.

My high school years were spent at a similarly conservative boarding school in Montreal, Quebec. This institution also produced few college-bound graduates, and many students had no realistic hope of going on to a secular higher education because of the poor foundation they had received in non-Jewish academic subjects. Graduates were relatively unprepared for taking SAT exams or for the rigors of higher education in subjects such as mathematics, history, literature, or science.

There was precedent, though, in my home for seeking a college degree. I certainly wanted one, even though my teachers at the yeshiva and my classmates decried it as a waste of time and energy. To my parents' credit, they actively supported my decision to leave the yeshiva world and, belatedly, seek a sound secular education. But then, they had known for a long time that I was uncomfortable within Orthodox Judaism.

At the age of eleven, a momentous thing happened to me: I discovered science fiction. The very first science fiction novel I read was Robert Heinlein's *Stranger in a Strange Land,* and in it I found a structure that enabled me to start fashioning my own questions about religion and my place in Orthodoxy. What a revelation—for the first time in my life I experienced a feeling of deep intellectual connection. It elated me: here was someone who thought the way I did. By the time I was thirteen, I had read everything of Heinlein's and had gone on to Isaac Asimov, Arthur C. Clarke, and Carl Sagan. I also branched out into general literature and discovered John Steinbeck, starting with his novel *The Pearl.* Through these tutors, I studied secular philosophy, science, and literature. I thrilled to the science that Asimov, Clarke, and Sagan revealed to me, and even more to the philosophy of Heinlein, whose books seemed to me exquisite essays on the human condition. Steinbeck opened my mind and heart to the joys of shared experience. These authors gave me the courage to question and stand up for my inner beliefs, which were at odds with those of the community in which I was living. I became particularly devoted to so-called "hard" science fiction, which became for me a guilty pleasure, my refuge from the world, my home away from home.

Flush with newly expanded horizons from these books, I was beginning to feel that the Orthodox view of the world was increasingly narrow—so Biblically oriented that it didn't even take into account actual Jewish history, let alone world history after Biblical times. Most graduates of my yeshiva would have been hard pressed to tell you when in history Moses must have lived, or what daily life had been like for people in that era; we understood nothing of the life of nomads in the Mosaic era, for instance. Judaism and history were taught as a single interwoven entity, with little or no references to non-Jewish culture or to concurrent events in the world that did not interact with Jewish culture. For example, although I was taught the writings of Maimonides, I was never permitted to learn the fact that in addition to being a renowned Jewish scholar, Maimonides had been a physician to Egyptian royalty in the twelfth century, and that the reach of his writings extended far beyond Judaic studies and influenced thinking in the non-Jewish world. Nor did I learn in yeshiva that leading rabbis of his time considered Maimonides a radical, viewed his works as heresy, and denounced him to the Inquisition.

Around this time, I began questioning my teachers and parents about basic tenets of Orthodox doctrine, though I quickly learned to do such probing in a careful manner, for while rigorous debate was supposedly a welcome mainstay of the Talmudic lifestyle, in practice acceptable debate topics were limited to those entirely within the belief system. It was fine, in this schematic, to spend all day arguing about the order of sacrifices in a temple that had been destroyed two thousand years ago—and, believe me, we spent many days doing just that—but raising the question as to whether animal sacrifice was divinely decreed or just a man-made form of worship was not fine at all; it was tantamount to heresy and not to be tolerated.

In the strict Orthodox community, censorship abounded. Magazines, television, movies, most fiction, and many other forms of literature and art were completely banned from our reading and viewing.

You were at risk of being expelled from school if you were caught peeking. Today this ban extends to the Internet.

Increasingly sensitive to the constraints put on my general learning by my religious upbringing, I simultaneously became aware that my feelings about that upbringing were different from those of most of the people around me. They seemed to want to remain in the culture; I wanted out. The revelation that I must leave was complete and fundamental for me, and I never changed my decision about it, though it would take another decade and a half, until I was twenty-seven, before I had finished extricating myself fully from the Orthodox community.

Many times during those years, I felt as though I were conducting a masquerade, displaying all the outward accoutrements of Orthodox Judaism but without the inward conviction. I was certainly not rejecting Judaism or God, but rather an Orthodox fundamentalism so rigid that in recent years I have referred to it (though only in jest) as Taliban Judaism.

Despite my misgivings about this masquerade, I continued to be a dutiful student at the yeshiva and learned a great deal there that was of use to me at college and, still later, in my profession. Perhaps most important, among all the things I learned in those years, was a set of fundamental skills: how to ask questions; how to acquire and analyze information—to deconstruct things; and how to be logical and follow the truth wherever it might lead.

At some level, my parents were aware of my struggles in the yeshiva learning environment. And so, with their blessing, I applied to and was accepted into college. I was fortunate to get in since I had virtually no background in the sciences or other secular studies. In fact, I had to spend two summers taking courses and passing five New York State Regents examinations in those courses, a prerequisite for obtaining a New York State Regents diploma. Without such a diploma, you did not have much hope of attending a four-year college in New York State.

While at college, I decided to become a physician assistant (PA), and after four years of undergraduate work, I entered a PA program. That program would lead me to a professional degree, though not to a master's. Today, many PA training programs are given only on the graduate level—you enter them after first acquiring a bachelor's degree, and when you graduate the program, it is with a master's degree or its equivalent. I think that's a better way to do it. A PA needs to be a bit older, to have more schooling under his or her belt before starting to work, because the responsibilities he or she faces as a new PA are immediately so great—caring for patients in hospitals and clinics, with only minimal supervision—that they demand not only a solid foundation but also a certain maturity that comes only with age and experience.

I enjoyed every minute of PA school. Raised on a steady Talmudic diet of such obscure subjects as learning what to do when your neighbor's ox falls into a hole on your property, I finally had course material into which I could sink my intellectual teeth.

PA school is like an abbreviated and accelerated version of medical school. Instead of attending, say, 120 hours of lectures in anatomy, we got 60. Instead of two years of didactic (theory) courses, as were offered in medical school, we took one; and instead of spending the ensuing two years in clinical rotation, we spent one year on hospital wards. The entire course of study for PAs usually amounts to a solid twenty-four to twenty-eight months of work and classes; the precise mix depends on the school, but all such training heavily emphasizes the *clinical* aspects of medicine. The training can be so relentlessly clinical because most people who become PAs do not go on to medical research. Another reason that our training spends less time on the underlying science is that a PA can practice only under the supervision—preceptorship—of an attending physician. However, when legally supervised, we can diagnose and treat, prescribe medications, first-assist in surgery, and so on, just as a medical doctor (MD) can. We can even sign prescriptions, hospital charts, and orders. The regulations delineating the scope of practice for PAs vary from state to state, sometimes considerably. Some states insist that charts signed by a PA must be countersigned by a physician within twenty-four hours, while others require such charts to be signed within a week or within a month.

While newly minted MDs go on to residencies and other postgraduation training—highly structured clinical training programs that can last from three to seven years—there is no similar requirement for PAs to go through a residency; you graduate, pass the national board exam, and then you're officially a licensed PA. Instead of a residency, PAs learn on the job, which allows them to put their classroom learning to immediate use. This also allows a PA to start earning money immediately, which was important for me because during PA school, I had married, and by graduation, our first child was on the way.

In the late 1980s, a young PA was a great thing to be. We were in tremendous demand, each graduate having a choice of about seven jobs waiting on the outside. During the last few clinical rotations of my training, physicians I had never met before would approach me in hospital locker rooms or hallways and give me their cards. "Call me as soon as you get licensed," they would urge, "I'm paying top dollar."

I chose as my first position a staff job with an inner city clinic located on Manhattan's Lower East Side that had its patients' fees paid mostly by Medicare or Medicaid. The clinic had never before hired a PA, but the director was a savvy businessman who realized he could pay a PA a third of what he would pay an MD but still get 90 percent of the work that a physician would do. His calculation made no difference to me; at the time, I was thrilled to have a $30,000 salary.

The clinic, as I had hoped, was a golden learning opportunity, giving me the chance to work with patients of all ages, from newborns to octogenarians, and providing constant traffic through the waiting rooms. There were few places in the city where I could have obtained as much hands-on and widely varied experience. I bought a new lab coat—full-length—several pairs of slacks, and a new stethoscope, and I plunged right in. My orientation at the clinic was short, as its directors firmly believed in the old med-school adage, "See one, do one, teach one." For three weeks, I was paired with and followed around one of the clinic's staff physicians, learning the ropes. After that I was turned loose on the patients, with a doctor nearby for supervision. And then, one week later, the doctor who had been supervising me was fired. It turned out that he'd provided false documentation when he was hired; though he'd been a physician in Russia, he'd neglected to obtain the necessary license to practice medicine in the state of New York; instead he had submitted to the clinic the credentials of a licensed doctor who had died some time ago. The clinic had to scramble to find someone else to supervise me.

That was my welcome to the unpredictable world of medicine.

The clinic had two "hard site" facilities, and we also provided services to a battered women's shelter and to a locked-down drug rehabilitation center. Once a month, our mobile van would pull up to a street corner, and we would offer services to whomever walked in the door. I never figured out how patients found that mobile van, since it seldom parked twice on the same corner—but they did, in hordes. We'd pull up, and the waiting room would instantly fill with people suffering from a dizzying array of maladies and displaying an equivalent variety of personalities and needs.

Of all the types of patients who made an impression, the most unusual to me were the prostitutes. After all, even though I was married and had fathered a child, I was still a somewhat sheltered Jewish boy from Brooklyn. You can imagine how flustered I was when my medical assistant told me that one of the prostitutes, a regular at the van, had a crush on me. I was teased unmercifully because this patient must have weighed three hundred pounds. Still, she was a very successful prostitute—at least, to hear her tell about it. Once, during a pelvic examination on this patient, I found a large green grape deep inside her vaginal vault. I couldn't resist asking her how it got there. She sighed and said, "I tole 'im, if he puts 'em in there, he better gets 'em all out." I declined to ask the follow-up question.

Practicing medicine alongside dedicated physicians and other staffers, I learned a great deal about providing care for the most indigent members of our community—for the shattered families and malnourished infants of the battered women's shelter, and for the unfortunates of the drug rehabilitation facility. Such places and patient populations gave me a glimpse into a world that served to wipe away some of the naiveté of this yeshiva boy.

Despite the array of experiences that the clinic afforded me, I decided to leave after only a year. Physician assistant salaries were absolutely exploding, and I had received offers that would almost double my current salary. The clinic really could not afford to pay me much more than it was doing, so I left, reluctantly but firmly, knowing of my growing family's needs. It had been a trying first year, but one that had seen me move from being a newly minted PA to becoming a blooded PA veteran.

From the Lower East Side, I went to Brooklyn to work for the Interfaith Medical Center, a facility run jointly by Brooklyn Jewish Hospital and St. John's Hospital. The Center was located in a pretty tough neighborhood and served a population similar to that of the clinic I had just left. I felt right at home.

My job was in the neonatal intensive care unit (NICU), which treated premature babies, some as small as 700 grams; we called them micro-preemies. The job was another eye opener. Once, I was doing a workup on a newborn for possible sepsis, or blood infection. The baby needed a spinal tap, a common enough occurrence in the NICU and something the PAs there did regularly. So I went upstairs to the maternity ward to find the baby's mom, to obtain her signature on the consent form for the procedure. Walking into the room, I saw a little girl laying on one of the beds, sucking her thumb. I asked where her mom was—and only then noticed her plastic armband. This thumb-sucking twelve-year-old girl was actually the preemie's mother.

At the NICU I saw firsthand the elements of one of the great debates raging in medicine and medical ethics today: the debate over the distribution of this country's precious medical resources. During my time at Interfaith, I watched a micro-preemie struggle to live for about seven months, during which time he had to undergo eleven surgeries, hundreds of cribside procedures, and countless sepsis workups—and then, tragically, die. His suffering was unimaginable, and his total health care costs, all borne by Medicaid, easily exceeded a million dollars. Yet even at the outset his chances of living had been less then one in ten, and, in the remote chance that he survived, he would most likely have been blind and profoundly retarded. Witnessing such circumstances raised crucial questions about whether the sheer expense of such an undertaking had been justified, and if it had not been, where we were supposed to draw the line in our efforts. These questions continue to haunt medical professionals around the country today.

Heartbreaking as the NICU sometimes was, there were plenty of happy moments that kept me going, and I would likely have stayed at Interfaith for quite a while, but eight months or so after I arrived, the hospital slipped into financial trouble and one of my paychecks bounced. I had to look for other work and soon found it at Beth Israel Medical Center in Manhattan. The man who hired me for the neurosurgery department at Beth Israel was the departmental chairman, a brilliant and somewhat wacky neurosurgeon. He was also the president of a private company that held a contract with a major group insurer, Health Insurance Plan of New York (HIP), to provide neurosurgery services (cranial, neck, and spinal) for the group's subscribers. I was paid a salary by the hospital and another by the surgeon for working at his HIP office. To this day, I'm not sure that the hospital ever learned about that second salary, but I certainly earned it by working more than eighty hours a week.

Neurosurgery was a large division of the hospital; the usual census on the neurosurgery ward was thirty-five to forty patients, and to care for them, the hospital had assigned four PA positions to the department. There were private patients and there were HIP patients; in those early years of managed care in America, the distinction between the two sets of patients on the neurosurgery floor was always obvious. Clinicians contracted with HIP for a flat fee per year, no matter how many patients they saw or operated on, giving them little financial incentive to perform surgery on the HIP patients (an essential idea of cost control in managed care). Not surprisingly I noticed that we tended not to do surgery on HIP patients if there was any doubt that they would benefit from the surgery. However, because private patients were paying individually for their services (usually through other insurers, of course), they tended to end up in the operating room regardless of any lingering doubts.

Our department didn't have house staff or residents (postdoctoral MDs), so the PAs did everything. I admitted patients, scheduled and prepped them for surgery, completed administrative paperwork, assisted in the operating room in the mornings, and then saw postoperative patients. All afternoon I changed dressings, administered tests, filled out discharge summaries, and wrote orders for patients who were going home. After grabbing a bite to eat for dinner, I'd spend the evenings reviewing the outpatient CT (computerized tomography) scans, myelograms, and MRI (magnetic resonance imaging) scans, determining who would be admitted next.

Drawing on my NICU experience, I quickly became one of the only PAs in the hospital who performed spinal taps, called on frequently when other hospital staffers had a patient who was a "difficult stick." After doing a spinal tap on a 700-gram micro-preemie, performing an adult spinal tap was as easy as steering a Mini Cooper into the Lincoln Tunnel.

Urged by my supervising physician to push my practice to the limit allowed PAs by law, I performed other procedures usually done by physicians themselves—procedures that, when I did them, often raised eyebrows. Once, in the surgical intensive care unit (SICU), I stuck a 60cc syringe into a patient's brain through a surgical incision we had made that morning. As my boss coached me over the telephone, I drew off some cerebral spinal fluid, thus relieving the pressure that had been building in the patient's brain. The procedure worked and the patient was fine, but a few hours later the SICU director found out what I had done and had a colossal fit. He complained to the hospital administration, and the subsequent brouhaha caused quite a flap. Everyone began weighing in and taking sides. Such a bedside procedure would normally have been done by a skilled neurosurgeon—but instead I had done it while being instructed by my supervising doctor, and the procedure had indeed been successful. After a few days, things cooled down, and I continued to practice as directed—on the edge.

My days at Beth Israel began at 5:30 A.M. and did not end until 8:30 P.M. Since I lived only a few blocks from the hospital, I was called at all hours to return to the hospital and do something that couldn't wait until the morning or until Monday. The amount of work I did and the variety of that work and its importance within the medical system demonstrated that PAs could be better used in our medical system, to take some of the burden from physicians, possibly bringing down the overall cost of health care. It doesn't really require a licensed MD—a person who has had four years of college, four years of medical school, maybe five more years of residency—to give an injection, perform a basic test, or do much of the other basic work of medicine. There is an adage in medicine that 90 percent of the time you draw from 10 percent of your knowledge; the other 10 percent of the time, you need to draw from the other 90 percent of your knowledge. Practically speaking, this means that 90 percent of the time the presenting problems of patients are *routine*, the sort of problems that PAs are well trained to cope with. If PAs did more of the 90 percent, routine sort of work, it would leave the MDs to concentrate on the 10 percent, the more complex and difficult matters.

At Beth Israel, my crazy schedule and relentless workload affected and exhausted me; I was further depleted because in addition to my paid work, I was attending law school at night. Relatives of mine had convinced me that if I added legal training and knowledge to my PA degree and expertise, I could clean up monetarily, perhaps specializing in medical malpractice.

The first year of night law school cured me of that idea. I hated what I was learning. There wasn't a branch of law that appealed to me in the slightest. The study of law was boring and, well, legalistic, rather than dealing with lofty principles and great ideas. Or perhaps I was being too harsh; I hadn't really wanted to go to law school, but I had attended because I thought it might indeed be interesting to merge medicine and law. I stayed long enough to understand that law wasn't for me. In particular, I was revolted by the notion of engaging in medical malpractice law.

Attending law school wasn't a complete waste of time because it enabled me to discover within myself a latent interest in all things forensic. I noticed an Office of the Chief Medical Examiner (OCME) advertisement in the *New York Times*, for PAs to work as MLIs. Intrigued, I considered applying, but was initially discouraged by the relatively low salary being offered. Then, on a rare free Sunday evening, I attended an opera recital at Carnegie Hall—and over the course of the concert, my beeper went off fifteen times (on vibrate). Fifteen times I had to go out into the lobby and use the pay phone to call the hospital. After the tenth such call, coming back to my seat, I thought to myself, "If your patients were *dead,* Shiya, you could probably sit through a concert without interruption."

That night clinched it for me. I applied for the chance to become an MLI for the OCME, and during my interview there, I was accepted for the position.

It was love at first sight. After learning what it was I would be doing, and why, I concluded that PAs were born for such a job. During my interviews for the position, I learned that the new chief medical examiner was staking his reputation on an innovative program in which PAs would comprise the entire investigative staff—and that therefore we would have all the support in the world. Moreover, even though I would be taking a serious cut in base salary, I was assured that I'd make out okay because there were too few investigators to handle all the work, so there would be a lot of overtime. I did the math: time-and-a-half meant that I could make in sixty hours what I'd previously had to work eighty to obtain—and sixty felt like a breeze to me after what I'd been through at Beth Israel. That was important to me, because now my wife and I had two children. I was twenty-five years old, thoroughly disenchanted with the Orthodox Jewish lifestyle, and with a marriage that was showing signs of crumbling. In that scenario, a new job carried the potential to turn my entire life around.

Quickly accepted for the MLI training program, I reported for work at OCME. In September 1990, I received my identification and my shield, emblazoned with the number 110 and the crest of the city. I was the tenth person employed in the program. But only seven MLIs, including me, were still working; the rest had already dropped out.

TWO

ONE DAY YOUR colleague Fred is in the office and he's okay. The next day he's absent, and you hear that he's ill; on the third, you receive an e-mail saying that he has passed away; on the fourth, you go to his funeral. At the wake, you gaze at Fred, laid out in a very comfortable-seeming casket. He actually looks pretty good, lying there in his nice suit and embalmer's makeup.

You may suspect that it's all set design and special effects, but you don't know the half of it. That casket has no real cushions; Fred's suit probably doesn't have a back. There is wadding stuffed up his nose and in his throat to keep fluids from leaking out, a plug in his backside for the same reason, and if he weren't wearing so much makeup he would look, well, dead.

Fred's travels as a corpse, and what happens to him along the path from the hospital to the funeral home, then on to the cemetery or crematorium, are unknowns to you—and you don't mind these matters being unknowns because dead bodies are taboo things, somebody else's problem. This isn't that different from the way we treat many other matters. We eat bread, but we don't grow wheat or know much about how it's grown; we wear shirts, but we don't grow, harvest, or spin cotton or sew the shirts ourselves. We just don't think about what goes into the process of getting bread to our plate or shirts on our backs. In much the same way, we may go to funerals, wakes, and cemeteries, but we don't deal with dead bodies. Instead we simply accept the sight of our friend, cousin, or spouse lying there in the casket, but give no thought to what went on behind the curtain so he or she could end up there. Many people who work in the industry, including MEs, funeral directors, and embalmers, do so because they wanted a peek behind the curtain. And they desired that peek because they are fascinated with death.

Death is still, cold, quiet, and gray. Life is moving, warm, noisy, and full of color. The opposite of life is not only death, it is also the absence of joy—which is why, sociologically speaking, the opposite of a funeral is a wedding. Though it was this fascination with death that led many of us to the industry, in reality our days are filled not with death itself or the struggle to know death, but with cleaning up *after* it. By the time we get involved with a body, death has come and gone, leaving us with only the empty shell, the abandoned luggage of what was once a human being. This is a key concept for those of us who deal with death's remnants on a daily basis; it's an understanding that we must have if we are going to do our work properly. Death merely heralds the beginning of our work.

Trainee medicolegal investigators (MLI-Is) definitely have to reach this understanding, and they do so not through gentle coaxing but through a rigorous sink-or-swim training program implemented by the more seasoned investigators at OCME. In my case, it began with my training officer telling me, during my first week on the job, that I would do the honors on the first body I ever saw at a death scene.

I didn't want to touch that first body. It was in awful condition and in exceedingly awful surroundings: a man of about sixty years of age in a single-room occupancy hotel on the Bowery, his emaciated body lying half-on and half-off a narrow bed in a filthy, roach-infested room barely large enough to contain the bed, a small dresser, and a chair. For the last twenty years of his life, this man had been a dedicated alcoholic, and the small sad room had been his home for most of those years. Some time before death he had defecated in his pants, and from the looks of his clothing, he had also regularly urinated on himself.

It was a sweltering September day in Manhattan, and the stench in that little room was so thick you tasted it. The foul miasma was compounded by contributions from the fifty or so other rooms on the floor, each housing another sad sack, none of whom seemed to bathe any more regularly than my guy.

I didn't want to go near him, let alone touch him, but I had to. My training officer stood just outside the door—there was no room for both of us in that room anyway—grinning from ear to ear as he watched me prepare my gear. I pulled out my camera and my clipboard, and as I put on my gloves, I said, aloud, "I can't believe this is *my* job." My words were uttered not in anticipatory glee or in regret, just in astonishment that this was something I could do—and was going to do.

Society needed me, or someone like me, to touch him. *You* needed someone to touch him, to find out what had happened to him, to verify who he was, whether he had any communicable diseases, and if his death in any other way might impinge on public health. And he needed someone to touch him because every dead person has a right to be examined, to learn whether foul play or bad treatment has brought an end to his or her life.

This man's body was particularly disgusting. There was a maggot infestation at his crotch that, I could tell, had begun even before death, birthed by professional-grade bad hygiene. I held my breath and got to it. Hesitant and awkward, I tugged tentatively at the body, glancing repeatedly at my training officer for guidance. My skin started to crawl because a cloud of body lice appeared when I disturbed the body. The maggots writhing under the decedent's skin made me slightly queasy. But I got through the task of investigating the body, which, of course, was just what my supervisor had hoped for—and with that one inspection I officially moved behind the curtain, becoming a participant in the elaborate play that would eventually deliver Fred into the scene in the funeral home which you attended as a mourner.

That first encounter as an MLI-I with a dead body, which we classified as a natural death due to chronic alcohol abuse, was also, as I would later realize, the beginning of another, intensely personal journey for me: to the state of mind in which I could honestly avow that I do my job because I love it—not because I love decomposing bodies, but because I have a highly developed fascination with death. We all share that fascination, at least to some extent, I believe, as evidenced by the tremendous popularity of television shows like *Law & Order* and *CSI*, though perhaps we in the ME's office do have more of it than civilians do. This fascination is what draws recruits to the death industry like moths to a flame. Death is the final unknown, and it is also unknowable. It is the ultimate mystery, and to me that makes it an irresistible challenge.

And so I got used to putting my hands on dead bodies, moving past the "ickiness" of the job in stages, just like most of my colleagues. I came to believe that anyone who was able to plunge in without any difficulties was someone I didn't want to share an office with, because that person inevitably turned out to be a sick puppy. Despite the way in which the people in the ME's office are portrayed by the media, we are not the sort who eat bananas in the autopsy room while cutting up a body or otherwise act creepy. Society projects its discomfort with death and dying onto my colleagues and me and enjoys portraying us as ghoulish. It's not true: most of my colleagues at OCME are warm, caring, and gentle and could make more money on the outside. They remain at OCME not because of a morbid fixation, but because they believe in its mission: uncovering the facts behind the death.

While always teaching me to be respectful of the dead, my profession also gradually conditioned me to see each new dead body not as a recently living individual, but as an artifact—a tangible item like the pill bottle on the desk at the death scene or the blood spatter on the wall—that can be evaluated by me in the same manner and for the same purpose that I examined the pill bottle and the blood spatter: to discover what had happened to the dead person. It's not lost on me that this body was once a person, but the person has left, and all I have to deal with is the corpus of what used to be a human being. It took three months for me to become comfortable around dead bodies, six months for the bodies to become artifacts, and a year for me to reach the point where I was able to attach no more emotional importance to the body than to the blood spatter on the wall.

In other words, during our first year, we MLI-Is learn to cope. The most important element in that coping is the growing understanding of our sense of duty—the obligation to do certain things that would be distasteful to you and almost everyone else on the planet. Every day, we MLIs take our fears out of their hiding places, examine them, and come to terms with what they have to say. It takes a special kind of fortitude to willingly confront and interact with a rotting body, or one that is cut up into pieces. And it takes a person who understands the social necessity of this act to do it properly.

There was much more to the job than I had imagined. My visions of rapidly becoming a younger version of Jack Klugman's *Quincy* were soon dispelled, for I had much to learn. My training would not only entail acquiring a tremendous fund of forensic expertise but also learning the agency's rules, regulations, protocols, and the subtle nuances of the political minefield that is New York City's civil service.

Around seventy thousand people die each year in New York City, and they die in every conceivable location—at work and church, in stores and parks, on subways and buses, in restaurants and theaters. Most people, though, die at home or in hospitals, or, to be more accurate, they are declared dead at a hospital. Their demise may have begun in a thrift shop on Bleecker Street, but continued during their travels to, say, the emergency room at St. Vincent's Hospital, where they finished the task of expiring.

More than a third of the city's yearly toll of deaths will be reported to the ME's office because they match certain criteria and therefore fall within our jurisdiction. To handle the volume, our office maintains a headquarters in Manhattan and satellite offices in each of the four outer boroughs. All of our training and educational programs take place at the main building, which, in addition to serving as Manhattan's borough office, houses the agency's citywide administrative functions and all of its laboratories. Very high-profile cases, such as the death of a politician or celebrity, or the victims of a mass fatality incident—even if the deaths occur in an outer borough—are often brought into headquarters. There is also a longstanding tradition that a police officer or firefighter killed in the line of duty anywhere in the city is brought to the main office in Manhattan for autopsy. It's not that the borough offices are inferior in any way; it's just that with the administration located in Manhattan it's easier to handle media interactions and special situations there.

The main office, that uncommonly ugly building at the corner of Thirtieth and First, sandwiched between two of the largest hospitals in the world, New York University Hospital and Bellevue Hospital Center, is always filled with activity. When I began, I was assigned for training to a PA and supervising MLI who had worked in that capacity with Dr. Hirsch before they came to New York City, when both were in the Suffolk County ME's office. He took me on an orientation tour of headquarters, and his running commentary gave me some understanding of the overall functions of the OCME. The administrative offices, medical records unit, communications and identifications units, and MLI squad room were on the first floor; the autopsy rooms and walk-in body refrigerators were in the basement; the MEs' offices were on the second and third floors, along with an employees' lunch room (three decrepit vending machines, two moldy sofas, and a battered table), and the information-systems department. The fourth and fifth floors held the toxicology, histology, and serology laboratories, and the photography unit. The sixth floor was a shambles, in the process of being renovated to accommodate the serology lab, which was changing its name to the forensic biology lab and expanding to take the entire floor. Everyone was excited about the newfangled testing involving DNA that was going to push the new forensic biology lab to the forefront of forensic science and criminal justice.

By the time we descended again to the first floor and the communications unit, my head was spinning, but my tutor insisted that I pay attention in the communications area, because "this is where it all begins; this is where the cases come in." In a relatively small room, clerks manned the phones 24 hours a day, 365 days a year, recording all the cases reported to OCME citywide. Most of the cases are reported by either physicians calling from hospitals or police officers calling from a death scene. Every once in a while a case gets reported by a funeral director or some other authority that has a body and requires our help.

The clerks seemed to be a surprisingly happy bunch, considering that every time their phone rang it was a call about someone being dead. At the time, the procedure required the clerks to write up the "Telephone Notice of Death" on multi-sheet carbon-paper forms—it would be years before computers entered the building. They recorded basic demographic information about the dead person and preliminary information about the case, such as the address where the body was found, who found the body, and who reported the death. A case number was issued and the case was assigned to an MLI.

The investigators served as the gatekeepers for the agency, performing a sort of triage, and just because a case had been written up by the communications unit did not mean there would have to be an autopsy, or even a lengthy investigation. I quickly learned that the MLIs separated the incoming cases into two main categories: hospital deaths and scene deaths. We dealt with each category in a different manner. Hospital deaths were almost always investigated entirely by telephone. The investigator would conduct one or more phone interviews with the reporting physician, who would present the case to the investigator. After the presentation, the investigator would then decide whether the body would require an autopsy or could be released. However, scene deaths (occurring outside of a hospital), which were usually reported by a cop calling from the incident location, often required an on-the-scene investigation, and the MLI assigned to these cases would spend most of the day out in the field.

In a small room adjacent to the communications unit was an office whose beat-up metal furniture looked as if it had been there since the 1950s. It was in this tiny room, the MLI office, that I learned how to do triage, to differentiate a case that needed to come in (an ME case) from a case we could investigate briefly and release (a No-Case), and from those we could decline to investigate at all (a Nonreportable). Wherever the body was, I learned the steps to take and the questions to ask of the reporting caller, using the caller's information to quickly discern the need for further investigation.

Society likes to group together similar things, to affix nice convenient labels so we can identify units as belonging to the same set. It's no different in death. Here society has developed a mechanism of grouping the many different causes of death into just a few categories subsumed under the title "manner of death." Such a grouping is needed because while there are many causes of death (countless, in fact) in New York we have decided that there are only six manners of death—six boxes into which all the various causes must be lumped.

There's a great deal of difference between cause and manner. In forensic terminology, the cause of death is the actual *disease* or *trauma* that took the person's life, while the manner of death refers to the *circumstances* by which the cause arose. In New York City, these circumstances are lumped into six manners of death categories: homicide, suicide, accident, therapeutic complication, natural, and undetermined. For example, if John is shot in the head, the *cause* of death is the gunshot wound to the head—any six-year-old child who has watched enough television is going to be able to make the correct diagnosis for that cause. The *manner* of death, however, is not so easily ascertainable. If someone shot John deliberately, the manner could be homicide. If John shot himself, the cause would remain the same, but the manner would now be suicide. If John had been cleaning his gun and inadvertently discharged the weapon into his head, the cause of death would still be the same, but the manner would be decreed an accident. If we couldn't figure out how John's gunshot was sustained, the cause of course remains the same, while the manner of death would be classified as undetermined. John's gunshot could not have arisen by therapeutic complication or natural manner, but it could have been by any one of the other four manners.

The key to doing triage with our incoming cases was learning to plug them into one of these six categories. Whether it was a scene investigation or an over-the-phone interview with a physician about a hospital death, the MLIs would first attempt to ascertain the cause and manner of death. Once we gathered as much information as possible, a disposition would be made. In the case of our friend John, because of the violence and the possibility of foul play, it would be ruled an ME case, meaning that his body would have to be brought in.

These tasks come right out of the city regulations. Section 557 of the charter of the city of New York states: "There shall be a medical examiner's office and it shall investigate all deaths of persons in the city of New York occurring from criminal violence, by causality by suicide, suddenly when in apparent health or in any unusual or suspicious manner." Additional rules governing what we do and delineating our areas of responsibilities are in the city's administrative code, Section 17-202, and in its health code, all of which empower us to conduct *independent* examinations of deaths that occur in New York City and fall within our jurisdiction. Independent means, for example, that we don't work for or answer to the police; we just do our job and come up with an independent finding that includes a precise identification of the decedent and our opinion on the cause and manner of the death.

We investigate, sometimes we autopsy, and in all cases, we write up a report that presents the OCME's best guess as to the cause and manner of death. Yes, essentially we guess, because when the ME's office issues a death certificate all we are doing is rendering our *opinion based on the facts available to us at the time.* Should important facts come up later, we reserve the right to alter our opinion and want to be on record in a way that allows for that possibility.

For the same reason, our records, meticulously kept by a staff of twenty, are held by law in perpetuity. Technically speaking, no case in our office is ever officially closed. During my early months at the ME's office, I enjoyed browsing through some of the really old record books, dating back to the early twentieth century. The causes of death listed therein seemed almost quaint. I read about people dying of the vapors and apoplexy, asphyxiating from exposure to illuminating gas or being trampled by horses. The records show that there certainly was a great deal of consumption going around back then.

35

It takes a staff of twenty to run the medical records unit because that unit also includes a very busy correspondence section. While our reports are not generally available to the public and not fully subject to Freedom of Information Act requests, they are available to certain individuals and institutions. The district attorney's office automatically gets a copy of every homicide file, and also may request a record if it is bringing or considering bringing a criminal case. A record is also available to the family of the decedent upon request as well as to the referring hospital, if the death occurred in that hospital. Should a criminal case be brought, a record would also be available to the defendant's attorneys, though, in that instance, only by subpoena. We also get hundreds of letters from prisoners demanding to see our records on their victims for their court appeals; we often must comply with those requests.

We need twenty people in the medical records unit for the same reason that we need forty MEs: New York City is filled with people, a certain percentage of whom die every day. By comparison, the Massachusetts ME's office has only five examiners to cover the whole state. Our office is unique not only in size but also in the way we divide the labor. Although OCME has about an equal number of MEs and MLIs, the former almost never go to a death scene, other than for training purposes. We MLIs handle all the investigations and all the death scenes. Unlike most forensic jurisdictions, our office is also a center of medical education, doubling as the Department of Forensic Medicine of New York University's medical school; Dr. Hirsch serves as chairman of that department. Through that NYU affiliation, our office graduates four board-eligible forensic pathologists a year.

Under Dr. Hirsch's administration, the OCME has become, in my opinion, the best medical examiner's office in the country. One of the reasons for this success is that it employs PAs as MLIs, who serve as its eyes, ears, and first examiners of bodies and death scenes.

On the whole, our office is a dynamic place, with scores of visiting physicians, aspiring MEs, medical and PA students, and paramedics rotating through for training each year. The turnover among MLIs is small but noticeable, today amounting to 5 percent every two years. But in the early 1990s, when I began, the loss rate was higher because the MLI corps had not been in existence very long and some PAs were picked for it who either decided after a while that they didn't really like the work, or who in the eyes of the supervisors weren't up to snuff.

The arc of training for an MLI-I can be best understood as a progressive role reversal. At the outset, the supervisor does most of the investigating and the trainee observes; by the end of a year of training, those positions are reversed, and the trainee does the bulk of the investigating while the training officer observes. In between those two points, the shift of responsibility is gradual and less readily categorized. As in all such shifts of responsibility, the trainee learns by doing, which means that he or she learns, in part, by making mistakes.

I certainly made my share.

As a trainee, I once entered a death scene in which a young woman lay on a bed, in the fetal position, with her hands together, positioned as a cushion for her head—the classic sleeping position, as you might pantomime it for a friend. There was dried blood across her wrists and pooled beneath her hands. The uniformed cop on duty and the detectives were speaking of her death as a suicide, and I quickly decided that they were correct: the decedent must have slit her wrists.

My supervisor leaned in toward the body, put on a thin pair of latex gloves, and through the glove, with his fingernail, scraped away the blood from one of the wrists. It came off readily, and underneath it there was no wound. "Shiya, it's pulmonary edema," he said to me of the dried bloody fluid, and traced it back from whence it had come: her nose. The blood was a flux that had emerged during her last moments and had then coursed down the face and over her hands and wrists. In a person as young as this decedent was, that finding almost always means just one thing: drugs. We searched the rest of the apartment, and soon enough found the drug paraphernalia that we were certain had to have been there. Later we made the determination that her death was due to an accidental overdose of heroin.

I learned several lessons from this mistake. First, I must not yield to the drumbeat of what others in the room were telling me about the death; rather, I must conduct my own investigation and do so with an open mind. Second, when there was blood evidence, I must go beneath the surface appearance to determine its source. The third lesson was less obvious: I needed to formulate a style of investigation in which I did not go near the body until after having thoroughly searched the periphery—had I followed that philosophy in this case, I would have seen the drug paraphernalia first, and would therefore not have made an easily refuted guess about the cause of death.

Eventually, for handling scene deaths I would adopt a variation of the classic crime scene investigation pattern, a way of approaching the body through making concentric circles around it, of an ever smaller diameter—indoors it would be in concentric squares, really, since most rooms are more square than round. I would start at the outer periphery and work my way inward, so that I only arrived at the body itself after I had reached an understanding of the context in which it lay.

In a similar fashion, I learned to do witness interviewing and fact gathering before examining *anything*. Once, a few moments after I had arrived at a scene, I was asked by a detective how long I thought the body had been lying there. Only a few months on the job, and not yet humbled by the mistake I was about to make, I glanced at the body, which was quite bloated, and blithely opined, "At least a week." The detective dutifully wrote this down in his little notepad and soon left. I finished my scene investigation and only then thought to talk to the doorman about when he had last seen the decedent alive. To my chagrin, the doorman stated positively that he had seen the decedent alive three days before. A little further investigating proved he was correct. We found an ATM receipt indicating the decedent had been outside three days before he died.

The apartment in this particular case was very hot, and had I known during my scene investigation that he had been alive and kicking three days before, I would have easily recognized that the decomposition I noticed had been heat-accelerated. Making the call to that detective to correct my time-of-death estimate was embarrassing, but it helped cement my habit of gathering all available information before I started poking around—and certainly before I began rendering opinions.

Many lessons devolved from the following instructions, cautions, and needlings that were said to me during my training—phrases that, in later years, I would find myself repeating to the MLI-Is whom I would train:

"Don't step in that."

"Put on your gloves before you touch anything."

"Don't put on your gloves until you've taken photographs."

"Turn the body over *away* from you."

"Aren't you going to look closely at those medicine bottles?"

"I didn't like the way you spoke to the family."

"The way you described the apartment in your report is not complete. You forgot to mention the rotting garbage smell in the kitchen."

During my early months of training, the senior MLIs supervising me at scenes were constantly correcting me. Once, I was about to let a family leave the death scene without obtaining important information from them. Another time, I forgot to ask the family to sign certain important forms. Other rookie mistakes included stepping in places that I shouldn't have. Like into a pool of blood on the ground in an outdoor death scene, just after I had bought, and was wearing, a new pair of white sneakers. I left a footprint outlined in blood here, a similar pattern there, and bloody tracks all over. The detectives investigating the scene had to be alerted to my misdeed so that they did not immediately put out an APB for a Reebok-shod killer—not to mention that I had murdered a perfectly good pair of eighty-dollar sneakers.

Another thing I had to learn at scenes was to curb the natural inclination to let my imagination run amok. I arrived at another early case, a triple homicide in Brooklyn, and began working the scene. Prior to looking at the bodies, I spent a half hour trying to reconstruct, from the trail of blood, and from the disarray in the apartment, what must have happened—how the three homicides had gone down. I did not realize that the other officials at the scene were getting increasingly frustrated. Finally I was pulled aside by an old Jewish crime scene detective, a cop for thirty-five years, with twenty-five of them in crime scene investigations. Outside the apartment, this guy told me two things.

"Listen, boychick," he said, "You seem like a nice kid, so I'm gonna give you some advice you should take with you for the rest of your career. First, you've been engaging in 'mental masturbation.' (What he meant was that I had been trying to figure out what happened, rather than tabulating what I'd seen.) That might be of some interest and pleasure to you, but it's of no help to anyone else in the room."

After this rebuke, I was careful not to let my imagination run ahead of the facts, and I spent my time gathering those facts.

When the old crime scene detective saw that I was taking the first lesson to heart, he offered another (it had little to do with the immediate case at hand, but he felt it was important to impart):

"Always look up at the ceiling at a crime scene; you'll be a real star."

The veteran had noticed that almost no one looked up at a crime scene investigation, but he thought that all investigators should.

Once I had mastered the basics of how to move around at a death scene without wrecking the place, and had figured out how to get through a basic death investigation, things started to go a lot smoother. I was still being corrected, but not as often. Though I was still making mistakes at scene deaths, they were mostly a result of being too cautious. In OCME terms, being overly cautious meant bringing in a body for an autopsy when it could well have been released to the family without one. As a trainee, I didn't want to screw up, so I thought it was wise to be cautious and ended up sending in just about every body I came across, unless it was a crystal-clear natural death. Even then, I would try to talk the family into an autopsy; I was terrified of missing something.

Gradually I realized that it takes courage to release a body to the decedent's family without having had it brought in and examined by a more senior medical expert. Nevertheless, gaining this confidence, and being able to make that essential decision without personal agony or subsequent regrets, is part of growing into the job. An MLI receives a lot of encouragement from the MEs when he or she avoids making this particular mistake, because every case you don't bring in is a case the MEs don't have to autopsy.

One such "mistake" I really lived to regret was to bring in a murdered dog.

The dog had been shot in an apartment alongside his owner, a suspected drug dealer. Since both man and dog had been shot, we needed to know if the two victims had been killed with the same gun or with different guns. If the latter were true, then the cops would be looking for two shooters. So what if one of the dead was a real walking mop, the shaggiest, oldest part-sheepdog I'd ever seen, with gray dreadlocks? I had the dog and his owner brought in for autopsies, and during those autopsies, the bullets were extracted. They were from the same gun, a fact that the police and we needed to ascertain. Nonetheless, when I returned to the MLI squad room the next day, I found that my colleagues had hung a sign over my desk: ACE VENTURA, PET DETECTIVE.

The ribbing continued for a while. During the next month or so, when I was out in my car, the two-way radio would crackle and the dispatcher would inform me that there was a cat dead on 84th Street, or a parakeet in Washington Heights, and ask—because of my "special sensitivity"—did I want to handle these particular calls? This type of humor was a big part of the culture at OCME, and one of the reasons why I frequently remarked that the city's mortuaries were surprisingly fun and happy places to work. We even had a mascot, of sorts. Cindy, as we called her, was an ornate brass urn containing cremated human remains. This is the underlying story: A taxicab driver had found the urn in the back seat of his cab one afternoon, and, not sure what to do, took it to a local police precinct. He was told to take it to the ME's office. The driver, of Indian extraction, was quite upset at having to cart around the remains, and as soon as he had placed them on our reception desk, he fled, leaving us little information about the urn or its contents. Eventually, we did learn Cindy's true identity: She had been a child, a little girl, who had died of natural causes. We attempted to return the

41

"cremains" to the only living relative, a grandmother, but she refused to accept the urn. So Cindy became the MLI mascot, escorted to all our annual holiday parties. We all knew our work was quite serious, but when we were out of the view of bereaved families, a gently irreverent attitude toward the Grim Reaper was the norm.

Some of my rookie mistakes weren't entirely of a forensic nature. Once I received a call from a family member who wanted her brother's body exhumed, some five years after his death in a hospital, because of a dream she'd had the previous night. This elderly, crotchety woman kept me on the phone for half an hour as she told me that in this dream her brother had appeared to her and said he could not rest in peace because he had been murdered. I heard her out, promised her that we would look into the matter, hung up the phone, turned to my training officer, and said, "Boy, we sure get a lot of wackos calling here." Of course I had neglected to shut off the speakerphone; not only was my supervisor listening in but the caller also heard everything I said. That the little old lady turned out to be a psychiatric patient, and that there was no validity to her claim, did not diminish the cringe-making impact of this lesson. After hearing this story, Dr. Hirsch said to me, "You have my permission to say anything you want to a family member—just hang up the phone first!"

At this time, I was let in on a secret about the OCME main building: the firm belief among the old-timers of the office that our headquarters was haunted. Indeed, if any building in the city had a right to be haunted, ours did, holding so many dead bodies, many of whom had died violently. Our haunting spirits seemed to be technologically savvy because they manifested themselves primarily in the telephone system and the elevators. Our chronic and irreparable phone problems kept a Verizon telephone repair crew busy, full time. Phones rang by themselves; speakerphones went on when you didn't want them to, calls did not transfer properly, and so on. All of our elevators also acted strangely; in particular, the freight elevator at the rear of the building was inhabited by a spirit with a sense of humor, who liked to open and close the doors for apparently no reason. For a long time, this spirit was favorable to me, opening the elevator as I approached, though it would close as other people approached. Perhaps I was propitiating it properly. Later on, I must have offended Otis, as I called the spirit, or else he left to haunt another elevator, because in 1998 the doors stopped opening at my approach.

During my training, I learned that unnatural deaths usually made for complicated scene investigations but were no-brainer triage decisions: obviously the body would be brought in for autopsy. On the other hand, natural deaths presented the investigator with the opposite scenario. Fewer hoops for the investigator to jump through at the scene— a relatively uncomplicated scene investigation—but often a difficult decision on whether to release the body. At a scene death, that responsibility rests solely on the MLI.

A natural death scene was less difficult to conduct, but getting to the point of deeming it a natural death required a relentless effort on the part of the investigator to prevent himself or herself from doing so quickly, and continuing throughout the investigation to maintain a high index of suspicion. It was a constant battle to avoid being lulled into a false sense of security, into prematurely concluding that because everything looked so peaceful, this just had to be a natural death.

Part of our problem arises from natural and unnatural (violent) deaths receiving different levels of response from the various agencies charged with looking into deaths, including the police and OCME. When an unnatural death (of a human being) occurs, the authorities must attempt to answer seven questions: Who, What, When, Where, Why, How, and a second Who. The police are primarily concerned with the first Who—who did it, who killed the decedent, and the Why, the motive. The remaining five questions require input from the OCME to answer, including that second Who, who is this dead person. In practical terms, this means that when a natural death occurs, the police department's attention span is very short—only as long as it takes for the ME's office to verify the natural cause. Once the cops have been given the answer to the whodunit question—it was done naturally, which means no perpetrator—they lose interest. They are perfectly happy to leave the divining of the answers to the remaining six questions to the OCME, which means, initially, to the investigating MLI.

We learned how to answer those questions as we were trained at scene deaths and in handling hospital deaths, but, perhaps more basically, we also learned from the rigorous, wide-ranging didactic training course that we had to attend every afternoon. Although we might spend our mornings in the field on scene deaths, or in the MLI squad room handling hospital cases, beginning at 2:00 P.M. every day we had two hours of lectures on topics ranging from blood spatter interpretation to how to testify in court. Most subjects were taught by MEs and senior MLIs, but the lecturers also included anthropologists, toxicologists, DAs, defense attorneys, police ballistics experts, and fire marshals who taught us about arson investigations.

In that class, we learned about every conceivable way people could violently die. We attended lectures on thermal injuries, cutting injuries, ligature strangulation, manual strangulation, and positional strangulation. We learned about gunshot wounds: close contact and loose contact; entrance wounds and exit wounds; wounds caused by large caliber and small caliber weapons, and jacketed and soft-nosed bullets. We learned to spot a shaken baby and how to investigate a sudden infant death syndrome (SIDS) death. We saw photos of people who had been shot, stabbed, run over, hanged, electrocuted, burned, and drowned, or who had fallen from heights or been beaten to death. The smorgasbord of violence was only half the curriculum. Classroom training also included many hours in which natural disease pathology was discussed—good old-fashioned heart disease and cancer, alcoholic liver degeneration, obesity, diabetes, tuberculosis, and all the other diseases that will eventually get you if you manage to avoid a violent death. The line between life and death, I learned in those classes, is exceedingly thin. And the place where that realization hit home was the autopsy room.

THREE

ALL THE TRAINING we were receiving, out in the field and during the afternoon lectures, came together in the hours and hours we spent in the morgue, observing and assisting the MEs as they performed the ultimate lab test, the autopsy.

I wasn't exactly shocked by my first visit to the autopsy rooms at the OCME, having encountered an anatomy lab full of thirty to forty cadavers during my PA training. Back then, as a PA student, I was unprepared for the array of sights that I witnessed. Some of the bodies had their faces covered; others didn't. Some had their veins and arteries exposed, their muscles and organs carefully dissected out and labeled; others were more intact. All were embalmed, and the odor of formaldehyde was not only overwhelming in the classroom, it clung to you for hours after you'd been near the bodies.

In the anatomy lab, I learned to deal with the sight of death, but in the autopsy room, I learned about the smell of it, as it quickly became clear just how bad dead bodies can reek. The bodies in the OCME autopsy rooms were not embalmed, and as a result they produced other odors, sometimes far worse—the stench of decomposition and of rotting intestinal contents. These digestive system aromas taught me one thing for certain: when someone eats cheap, fast-food cuisine before they die, invariably they will stink worse after death than those whose final meal is macrobiotic.

An autopsy room is, in many ways, the mirror image of an operating room (OR). At the morgue, unlike in an OR, you gown up but don't scrub up—because you are protecting yourself, not the patient. For the same reason, afterward you make darn sure to scrub down, because the bacteria coming out of a dead body are very alive, and you need to make sure they all go down the drain.

The word *autopsia* in Greek means seeing for one's self. And that's what is done in the postmortem examination.

The layperson's attraction to the autopsy room, I believe, is the same as it is to a roadside accident—we like to slow down and look at the carnage. The larger field of forensics is itself fascinating, what with examinations of hair and fibers, microscopic traces of drugs and so on, but for attention grabbing the granddaddy of them all is the autopsy. Certainly the autopsy has more "ickiness" associated with it than hair and fiber analysis.

While this sense of ickiness and the thought of physically cutting into a dead body repulse most people, I maintain that it shouldn't. A great many times I've heard family members say, "Please don't cut him up. I don't want him to go through that after everything else he's suffered." Though this emotional response is easy to understand, it's not really logical. Not only is the cutting necessary to discern the truth about a given death, but it is not uncomfortable for the person who used to live in that body. The discomfort that exists is felt purely by the living as they think about the autopsy. The dead feel nothing.

This is not to say that cutting up a body is easy at first; indeed, to become professionally involved with autopsies at OCME, one must first reach the emotional point where he or she can incise bodies with impunity. To arrive at that mental place, it is essential to develop a mind-set that sees the body as an artifact, creating a sense of objectivity similar to how clinicians in the OR perceive and deal with an anesthetized patient. As I watched my more seasoned colleagues at OCME put on their scrubs and aprons upon entering the autopsy room, I noticed early on that they also donned (or crept into) a shell that permitted them to mentally detach themselves from emotional involvement, to handle traumatized remains without becoming traumatized. I quickly realized that, just as I had to learn to objectify decedents while performing scene investigations, it was now my task to develop an autopsy-room façade.

Though we death professionals work hard to cultivate our shells, we do not expect a family to have our level of objectivity, any more than a surgeon can expect cold logic from the family of a patient on whom he is about to operate. That's why one of our tasks is to keep the family's perspective in mind when we're discussing an impending autopsy of their family member. Some of us tried to gain that empathy by imagining that it was our loved one about to go under the knife; others, by just remembering how they felt while watching their first autopsy. This perspective is necessary in the family interview room; the shell cannot be present, or at least must be somewhat pulled back during conversations with families or else we will seem callous and inconsiderate. However, the second we walk out of the family interview room and proceed down to the autopsy suite, the shell must click right back into place. For in the autopsy room, a dead body must become a trove of evidence that may yield clues to its former inhabitant's demise. When we are determining which bodies to autopsy, the central question we ask ourselves is whether we'll learn anything from doing the autopsy on that particular body. If we think we will, then we have the body brought in and perform a postmortem. If we don't think we'll learn anything more than we have gleaned at the scene, then we don't have the body brought in.

Although generally any violent or unnatural death merits a trip to the autopsy room, families do have a right to object, particularly on religious grounds; we, in turn, have an obligation to attempt to accommodate their wishes when we can. Sometimes that is possible. In situations where the law does not mandate an autopsy, we can usually work it out with a family—for instance, if the case of suicide is very clear, from notes left behind and other clues, and if the family does not want an autopsy, we may be able to make our findings without putting a knife to the body. In addition, advances in technology have created more and more noninvasive procedures like CT and MRI scans that *sometimes* yield enough information on which to base a finding without having to autopsy.

Often a family that resists an autopsy will ask me a version of this question: "They put a man on the moon, and you're telling me that with all the technology that's available today, you still have to cut him up?" Essentially the family is demanding to know why we are not using a CT scan or MRI to find out what has gone on inside the body of their loved one, instead of doing a traditional autopsy. This is a very good question, and the old answer to it—because noninvasive means aren't precise enough to tell us what happened to the decedent—is changing.

In clinical medicine, the general purpose of CT and MRI scans is to limit the need for invasive diagnostic procedures, since the less you physically poke around inside someone, the greater his or her chance of getting out of the hospital alive and in one piece. Traditionally this concern was considered a nonissue once the patient was dead. After all, what harm can poking around do to a dead person? While at present even the very best imaging procedures available cannot rival the wealth of information that a skilled physician can gather by going inside the body, in the not-too-distant future, the balance between the information we can discover from actual samples and what we can obtain through noninvasive procedures may shift in favor of the latter. The grail for ME's offices might then be a virtual postmortem that could potentially yield equivalent, if not more, information than an actual autopsy, while sparing families from having their loved one undergo an autopsy that perhaps runs counter to their religious principles.

This would be especially useful when dealing with those autopsies that we are required by law to perform, regardless of objections. The following unfortunates receive automatic trips to the autopsy table: homicides, people whose deaths may involve threats to public health (such as outbreaks of plague, anthrax, or Legionnaires' disease), and prisoners. A prisoner, by the way, is defined as anyone incarcerated in a prison, remanded to a mental institution, or even just detained by the police at the time of death. Although the law absolutely mandates an autopsy in these cases, if the family objects, particularly on religious grounds, there are steps that we can take to ease their trauma. For example, some Buddhist sects do not permit the remains of the faithful to be refrigerated, so we try to autopsy those bodies quickly and release the remains to the family on the same day.

Similarly, special steps need to be observed when dealing with members of the Jewish population that require autopsy. Jewish tradition forbids autopsy and, further complicating things, demands that any blood spilled before or after death be interred with the body. Moreover, the burial must take place within twenty-four hours of death, and until the burial, a member of the faith must attend the body at all times. Given New York City's large Jewish population, the OCME quickly became expert in what we called the "rabbinical autopsy." When faced with a mandated autopsy on a Jewish decedent, a well-rehearsed routine would commence at OCME. Rabbis from various Jewish funeral homes would arrive and sit with the body until it was autopsied. The autopsy would be conducted as usual except that the entire procedure would be done with the body inside a waterproof body bag. This way, any blood leaking out of the body during the autopsy would be caught by the bag, which would then be buried with the body. At least one rabbi would attend the autopsy and supervise the collection of bloody paper towels or anything else produced during the autopsy that might have to be buried with the remains. The body would usually be removed to the funeral home by the rabbis immediately following the autopsy.

The willingness of OCME to go the extra mile to accommodate a family is not limited to highly religious Jews or to any particular sect or religious group. Any reasonable request by a family member is met with the utmost sensitivity, and every attempt is made to accommodate that family member's wishes.

Interestingly enough, the rationale for performing a mandatory autopsy on every homicide victim stems from the famous death of a rabbi. In 1990, Rabbi Meir Kahane, the founder of the Jewish Defense League, was murdered in New York, but because of religious objections from his militant religious followers, his body was not fully autopsied. Instead, a limited autopsy, a "bullet-ectomy," was done and most of the normal autopsy was foregone.

During the murder trial that followed, the defense attorney for El Sayyid Nosair, the man on trial for killing Kahane, accused the NYPD and OCME of a cover-up and of framing his client. On cross-examination this attorney tarred and feathered the ME personnel who testified for our office, primarily because a full autopsy had not been done. While there had been no conspiracy to frame anyone, the fact that a full autopsy was not done looked bad. After this case, the rule was firmed up: every single homicide would be autopsied, regardless of whether we'd learn anything from that autopsy, and regardless of familial or religious objections.

At the OCME, we begin autopsies at 8:00 A.M. and stop them only once the cases for the day are completed, which is usually by 12:00 P.M. A basic autopsy takes about an hour. "Any longer," quips Dr. Hirsch, "and you're not practicing medicine, you're holding services."

The whole process begins when you enter a brightly lit room that is surprisingly noisy, what with the sounds of saws, bolt cutters, doctors talking, and water running. In addition to the noise, it is also surprisingly hectic, since generally three or four autopsies are going on at the same time. There are eight autopsy tables laid out in a row, facing the sinks that line one fifty-foot wall of the rectangular room. On my first day, my training officer pointed the sinks out, telling me, "If you're gonna throw up, do it in the sink, *not* on the body. And also, take your mask off first or you'll drown." Indeed, it was advice worth heeding.

As you approach the first table, you see that the body is intact and laid out, naked and face up. While you were gowning up outside, its clothes were removed and external photographs were taken. The body was weighed and measured for height. With those logistics out of the way, the ME now notes any remarkable external features, such as deformities, amputations, lesions, trauma, tattoos, and the like. Careful attention is paid during the preliminary external survey to the eyes and inner eyelids for signs of petechiae, small spots of hemorrhage that can be an indication of trauma caused by strangulation or compression. The mouth is also carefully examined for the presence of lacerations to the inner lips, broken teeth, or any other subtle indications of trauma.

After the external exam is accomplished, the ME, taking up a position on the decedent's right side, grabs a scalpel and begins the internal examination. He makes a deep Y-shaped incision across the entire trunk: from the left and right collarbones down on two diagonals to the top of the sternum or breastbone, and then straight down the center line of the chest and abdomen all the way to the pubis bone. Then he peels back the skin and underlying muscles from this incision—we use the word *reflected* to describe this action. That exposes the ribcage protecting the heart and lungs, and the abdominal viscera (organs and guts), which are covered by the omentum, a fatty apron of connective tissue. Putting down the scalpel, the ME picks up a long bolt-cutter, the kind police use to snap locks. With this tool, he snips the ribs along the sides of the body, one by one, until he frees the entire front breastplate, ribs, and sternum. Then he lifts out and sets aside the ribs/sternum combination as a connected series of bones. The heart and lungs are thus exposed. The omentum is pushed aside, revealing the abdominal viscera.

Scalpel back in hand and reaching in with gloved hands, the ME then cuts out each organ and individually weighs, examines, and dissects it. The weighing is very important—one of the best ways to tell right off the bat if there is something wrong with an organ is if it weighs too much or too little. A normal, nondiseased adult heart, for example, weighs in at between 300 and 500 grams (about half a pound), depending on the size of the person in whom it used to beat. Certain diseases, such as high blood pressure, can cause the heart to grow dramatically larger, and this pathologic condition, called cardiomegaly, can kill you.

A famous case of cardiomegaly was found in the heart of André Rene Roussimoff, better known as André the Giant, a French-born American wrestler and actor. Roussimoff actually suffered from acromegaly, or gigantism. At the time of his death, he was close to seven feet tall and weighed over 500 pounds, and his heart reportedly weighed an amazing twelve pounds.

After the ME is done examining the heart, which includes cutting into the coronary arteries to look for plaque, and checking out the valves and chambers, he attends to the other organs. The healthy liver is a huge, red-brown, floppy thing that looks exactly like the raw calf's liver your mother might have brought home from the butcher when you were a kid. On the other hand, a diseased liver, like a cirrhotic or fatty liver that we find in alcoholics, or in ducks that are force-fed to produce foie gras, is often smaller than normal, yellowish, and stiff. You can spot an alcoholic's liver from across the autopsy room. Similarly, a smoker's lungs look drastically different from normal lungs. Dedicated smokers develop sooty deposits in their lungs that can turn lung tissue from a normal pinkish–blue-gray color to very black; in advanced cases, the lungs can become stiff and even develop large holes.

The stomach is filleted open, and the contents, if any, are examined. When I first began attending autopsies, I was disappointed that stomach contents were usually a tan- or gray-colored mush. From innumerable television crime shows, I had expected to see some easily recognizable remnants of the decedent's last meal. While some residue is occasionally visible, particularly from fibrous foods like broccoli or corn that remain more or less intact in the stomach for a long time, most often what we find in terms of stomach contents is no more than well-macerated mush.

Continuing down the digestive tract, the ME next "runs the bowel." A loop of intestines is grabbed near the point that the intestine joins the stomach, and the loop is punctured. An open scissors is inserted into the puncture point, and the bowel is pulled back against the scissors until it is entirely cut open, down to the rectum. This is, as you can imagine, a particularly smelly part of the autopsy. Not surprisingly, many MEs have their morgue assistants do the actual opening of the intestines, and they wait to examine the bowel until it has been washed.

Once the abdomen is done, it's on to the pelvis and its organs. During the autopsy of either sex, the rectum and anal sphincter are examined and the bladder is removed and studied. In males the scrotal sac is opened and the testes removed and sectioned. The penis is examined and the urethra (the tube running down its center, through which urine and semen travel) is swabbed. This swabbing can produce evidence of recent sexual activity or the presence of sexually transmitted disease (STD).

As with males, in females the examination of the genitalia and pelvic organs can reveal evidence of recent sexual activity, help us to differentiate between forced and consensual sex, and detect the presence of STDs. In women, the autopsy can also reveal if the decedent had ever borne children and if so, approximately when. During the autopsy, the ovaries, fallopian tubes, and uterus are removed, examined, and sectioned. The vaginal vault is examined, as are the external genitalia. If sexual assault is suspected, a so-called rape kit is used to swab (separately) the vagina, anus, and mouth with long cotton tipped applicators; any collected evidence is sent to the lab. If the decedent was raped as well as murdered, careful preservation of DNA evidence is of paramount importance, because in few other types of homicides do perpetrators leave such a clear calling card.

Throughout the autopsy, removed organs are sectioned, or to put it in layman's terms, "sliced up," on a cutting board, similar to the ones used in most kitchens. Small sections of every organ are carefully snipped off and placed in stock jars that are then sent to a storage room, where they are kept for at least ten years.

Samples of the blood, bile, urine, stomach contents, liver, brain, and anything else that the ME thinks appropriate to assay are sent to the toxicology lab to be tested for drugs and poisons. Often the ME will also elect to send vitreous humor—commonly known in the autopsy room as "eyeball juice"—to the tox lab. A long needle on a large syringe is pushed into the corner of each eyeball in turn, and all of the fluid is sucked out. This deflates the eyeballs. Sunken eyeballs would look terrible in an open casket, so the eyes are then refloated by injecting saline solution into them until they are once again nice and plump.

After the ME has finished examining the insides, the body lies on the table, empty of all of its organs; in the parlance of the autopsy room, it is a "canoe." The physician stuffs what remains of the viscera into a black garbage bag, and inserts the bag into the abdominal and chest cavity of the corpse, refilling the canoe. If necessary, the ME will then cut open and examine the insides of the four extremities. Most of the time, this is not done because the organs will have provided enough information on the cause of death.

The neck is then dissected and the tongue is pulled down and out through the hole under the neck and examined. (When drug dealers do this to an informant after they kill him, they call their procedure a "Colombian necktie.") As most mystery-novel readers know, at this point in the autopsy, careful attention is paid to the delicate "strap" muscles of the neck, and to the tiny hyoid bone that overlies the windpipe, especially in a case where strangulation is suspected.

Moving up to the brain, the ME makes an ear-to-ear incision in the scalp, at the level of the eyebrows but in the *back* of the head. Then he or she pulls the scalp forward—clean off the skull bone—over the eyes and face, down to the chin. Putting aside the scalpel, the ME takes up a whirring saw and uses it to cut off the top of the skull. The pate doesn't come off easily, so the ME will exchange the whirling saw for a sort of small chisel and use it to go around at the cut mark, prying up the skullcap. When the cap finally comes apart from the rest of the skull, there is a sucking sound like none other I have ever heard.

Now the ME takes up the scalpel again and goes around with it inside the cavity, using one hand to support the brain while the other (with the scalpel) severs the connective material that holds the brain in place within the skull. Once the brain is cut from its attachment to the spinal cord, it is ready to be lifted out. It is surprisingly gelatinous—like a soft-boiled egg—and to be properly examined, it must first be removed and hardened. The ME scoops the brain in gloved hands and drops it gently into a bucket of formalin, a pickling solution containing formaldehyde. The brain will then sit in the neuropathology room for the duration of the hardening process—making it into a hard-boiled egg—which will take about two weeks. After that, the brain can be sectioned, cut into small equal slices like bread in a bakery machine, and examined. If appropriate, small samples can be more minutely examined under a microscope. In our "Brain Room," there are shelves of white buckets containing human brains, and yes, one white bucket is labeled "Abby Normal."

After the brain has been removed and placed into the formalin, the autopsy is officially over. The ME calls for a morgue attendant who sews up the body cavity, using a large curved needle and heavy waxed twine. Wadding is stuffed into the skull where the brain used to be, the skullcap is replaced, and, using the same needle and twine, the scalp is sewn back on. The cutting has been done with precision and some delicacy, so that if a family desires it, the autopsied body can later lie in an open casket and not appear to have been cut into at all. Judicious placement of the head on a pillow will conceal the incision at the hairline in the back of the neck, and the other cuts can be hidden by clothing.

As mentioned earlier, the autopsy of an adult body, from opening to closing, generally takes under an hour. The exceptions to this rule are the complicated homicides, particularly multiple gunshot wounds because ascertaining the bullet paths and trajectories by means of long metal probes can be a tedious and time-consuming task.

I have heard MEs grouse when they are assigned a multiple gunshot wound case; the axiom is, "I would rather autopsy five bodies, each with a single gunshot, than one body with five wounds." It's not that the ME prefers mass murder, but rather that a multiple gunshot case can be incredibly complicated. Each bullet must be marked to ascertain its path through the body and direction of travel; entry and exit wounds must be identified. Every step must be fully documented, so that the procedure will be able to withstand blistering scrutiny from the defense, should the case be brought to trial. Often, the most crucial testimony offered by MEs involves the direction in which bullets were traveling—for example, in a "police shooting" case in which other witnesses contend that the decedent was shot in the back by police. It is crucial that the autopsy be able to confirm or refute the eyewitness testimony.

Once the autopsy is concluded, and while the attendant is busy sewing up one body and fetching another, the doctor dictates the findings or does other paperwork. When the next body is ready for autopsy, the doctor reappears in the autopsy room ready to start the process all over again.

Although the physical autopsy has ended, the OCME autopsy process is just beginning, because the doctor must then deal with the reports from the toxicology lab and do some first-hand tissue examination or microscopy. The entire process can take up to six weeks to finish and entails the doctor putting in, on average, about ten hours, what with the microscopy, paper reports, dealing with the family and family physician, and the like. But the bodies are not permitted to hang around with us for the full six weeks, and they are routinely released to families and their designated funeral directors within twenty-four hours of finishing the initial cutting and sewing-up part of the autopsy.

Physical findings from the autopsy are classified as A, B, or C. Class A are findings inconsistent with the continuation of life—they are conditions that if you have one or more of them, you can't be alive, such as a bullet hole in the heart or brain. Class B are findings of advanced disease or trauma; any one of these *could* kill you but not necessarily; however, a combination of two or more certainly suffices for a cause of death. In this class are things like atherosclerosis—you can't see it on the surface, and it is possible to have atherosclerosis and survive, but probably you won't if you have it in combination with, say, a blood clot. A similar combination of Class B findings in a traumatic death might consist of a moderate-sized subdural hematoma (bleeding on the brain), combined with a bruise on the brain, accompanied by swelling.

Class C findings are signs of disease or mild trauma that by themselves would not cause a person's death. If an autopsy turns up nothing at all aside from a few Class C findings, it is very likely that such a case will find its way to the "pending further studies" pile.

The more usual outcome of an autopsy, though, is that the findings will confirm the guess of the MLI, done at the death scene or during triage, about the cause and manner of death. Most of the time an autopsy simply dots the *i*s and crosses the *t*s of the MLI's on-the-spot investigation.

We once did a retrospective study of overdose deaths: Out of one hundred deaths that had been diagnosed at the scene as drug overdoses, the autopsy toxicology reports confirmed the opinion of the MLI at the death scene ninety-nine of the one hundred times as to the causative agent. This was an important finding because it gave MLIs in the field more confidence when voicing their opinions. If at the scene they suspected heroin, the statistics showed that they were likely correct. Knowing that your surmises are being validated in the autopsy and lab is a great help to an MLI.

One staple of crime dramas is the plotline in which the body is brought into the autopsy room with no outward signs of the cause of death. That's fiction—it is rare that at autopsy we find a cause of death that has no outward sign, or gave no premonition. Most of the time, when a body is brought in because the precise cause of death was not obvious at the scene, it leaves the autopsy room with a finding that the death was from "natural" causes that were simply not visible on the surface.

Moreover, once we are armed with the information on the natural cause obtained at autopsy, we are usually able to go back to the family and elicit corroborative data. For example, a forty-five-year-old man dies suddenly at work, but we are told at the scene that he has "no history" of heart disease. The autopsy finds that he had severe atherosclerosis. Later, when we question the family again, they now remember how the decedent had "indigestion" for the two weeks preceding his death—a fact they simply had not thought to tell the MLI during the investigation of the death prior to autopsy.

Medicolegal investigators are not only good at predicting overdoses, in general we're also good at predicting most causes and manners of death. If we say it's a natural death, it usually is, and the autopsy almost always comes to the same conclusion. While a regular device used in crime fiction is to have a body come into autopsy labeled as a natural death and leave as a homicide to be solved by the hero detective, in reality, this almost never happens. Since MLIs began to be the first-line investigators at OCME, not a single body has had to be exhumed from its grave on the grounds that we missed the real cause of death at the scene, during an investigation.

FOUR

DURING MY TRAINING year as an MLI-I, it wasn't only my supervisors and instructors who had to teach me. I learned lessons from cops and detectives, frequently when they weren't even trying to be teachers.

Such was the case with my first homicide. The decedent was a prostitute found by a jogger at the northern edge of Manhattan, under the Madison Avenue Bridge, along the banks of the East River. The Harlem River Drive, a major highway, runs above the site, and while passing motorists on that highway couldn't see the body, the Japanese tourists aboard the Circle Line sightseeing boat on the East River certainly could, and they nearly tipped the boat over when they all moved to one side with their Nikons to take a picture of a "typical" New York City scene.

It was clear to me, from my initial survey of the body and the location, that the woman had been killed elsewhere and dumped under the bridge. But as I continued working, the lead police detective went over to the decedent and stuck a handwritten note in her hand. It read, "I can't take it any more so I'm jumping off the bridge." And he accompanied the note with a grin at me and said, "Looks like a suicide."

"I don't get the joke," I said later to my supervisor, as we were in the car on the way back to the office.

"Cops don't like homicides," he explained. "There is just too much involved for them in working one." I expressed surprise; after all, like the rest of us in the United States, I had been brought up on a steady diet of popular culture crime stories in which characters like Kojak *lived* to catch killers. My supervisor shook his head at my naiveté.

Cops don't like to work murders, he suggested, because homicides mean they'll have to do too much paperwork. How much paperwork? Well, if the detectives were to fully fill out all the requisite "DD 5" forms—the basic report form of an NYPD gumshoe—on one single case, they would fill a book. Every witness to whom the detectives speak, every lead they follow, everything they do that is associated with their investigation of a homicide must be carefully documented. And even when the detectives are conscientious about doing their paper-work, another problem for them can arise—by filling out the forms they may have documented a misstep in their investigation, some small and insignificant thing, but one that a defense attorney could later blow up into a huge deal to make the detectives look like bungling amateurs. Consequently, among detectives there is a credo of paper-work avoidance.

A second set of problems for detectives who catch a homicide arises from the need to deal with a victim's family, and to do so over a period of months. As time wears on, if no progress is made on an investiga-tion, such families tend to get upset and to complain. Beyond these in-vestigative headaches, there can be political ones. Police bosses are under enormous pressure from city hall to keep the "numbers" (of homicides) low, and to solve or "clear" the murders that do occur. This dual pressure then gets translated downward to the precinct detectives.

For all these reasons, cops, especially detectives, have a natural re-sistance to concluding that a death scene is a homicide. We MLIs, how-ever, are not charged with preventing crime or directly with clearing cases and thus are immune to such pressures. We are taught instead to keep our "index of suspicion" high. I translated that edict into an inter-nal directive to "treat each death as a homicide until it was proven otherwise," and I repeated this mantra in my head at every death scene I walked into.

Slowly but surely, I was building in my mind a library of tech-niques, experiences, and tools that were making me into a better inves-tigator. As my knowledge of the profession deepened, I used my own gut instincts and refused to rely solely on the cops' side of the story. Years later, when I had become a more seasoned investigator, I was called to a "natural" death scene at an apartment in the Ninth Precinct, an apartment that had been illegally subdivided into smaller apartments. The action began as I stepped out of the elevator; a lone uniformed police officer, the only official person present, was standing guard at the apartment door. Walking around the hallway were quite a number of people, who I surmised were tenants of the illegal rooms, moving into and out of the apartment and just milling around. The cop didn't stop anyone else, but he brusquely asked me what my business was there. Amused, I pointed out that both my driver and I were wearing distinctive OCME windbreakers and had our IDs prominently displayed. He grudgingly allowed me to enter the milling crowd and the apartment, and I soon discovered that his dismal powers of observation were a portent of things to come.

As I stood just inside the doorway, a tall, cadaverously thin black man drifted over to me. He vaguely introduced himself as the decedent's husband. He seemed disoriented; I suspected he was high or had been using drugs for so many years that his brain had been fried. Slowly he led me to one of the many small rooms in the apartment, where a very emaciated black woman lay on a bed, dead. Though the small room was dimly lit, I could immediately see what I suspected were dried bloodstains on the bedding.

The cops, with their anti-homicide mind-set, had accepted the husband's explanation of the blood on the bed, which was that his wife had been menstruating. So satisfied with this explanation were the detectives that they had even left the scene before my arrival. Employing the lesson that I learned at that crime scene so long ago, I glanced up and immediately noticed a "cast off" blood spatter on the ceiling. All my internal alarm bells started clanging. I ushered the husband out and, with my driver holding a flashlight, conducted a closer examination of the body. This revealed that the decedent had been beaten and then strangled to death. She had ligature marks around her neck, some of her teeth had been knocked out, and there were lacerations inside her mouth. She also had a scalp wound under her matted hair.

This case really drove home for me the power of mind-set. I told the cop on duty to have the detectives come back to the scene, on the double, and while he was at it to summon the precinct's supervisors— and to detain the husband. When the detectives and their squad leader arrived, I told them I'd never heard of or seen projectile menstruation and pointed at the blood on the ceiling, which could not have gotten there from menstruation. That much was obvious, but even so, the cops—unbelievably stuck in their mind-set—tried to talk me out of my assessment that the woman had been murdered. Only after I had shown them her wounds, the real source of the blood spatter on the ceiling, did logic prevail, and they arrested the husband.

Keeping my index of suspicion high was a useful tool, but while I was developing it as an MLI-I, I had to learn to calibrate it. Early on, when entering a home, no matter how benign the scene within might appear to be, I viewed the decedent as a homicide victim and the family members present as potential suspects. Even if the decedent was a 101-year-old little lady lying on her bed, with a beatific smile on her face, and attended by loving, grieving family members, I saw a murder victim and a group of evil people who had knocked her off for the insurance money. During my first year, I slowly dialed back that inclination, until I was able to maintain a healthy amount of suspicion while not treating every family member like a mass murderer.

In fact, one of the most important understandings that I developed during my year of MLI-I training was that the *families* of decedents were really the clients of our office. Our first duty, of course, was to represent the people of the city in determining the circumstances of a death, but quickly I came to see that we also serve the family of the decedent in the processing of the death. Part of my task was therefore to enter a chaotic scene, in which a grieving family was confused and distraught, and to try to restore some semblance of order for them and guide them through the process of what happens to a body after death.

Dealing with the families at death scenes became an art form. I learned to consider relatives as suspects yet sympathize and empathize with them as well—since, after all, they just might turn out *not* to be killers. I was required to be firm yet gentle, tough yet kind, and in control of my emotions, yet not too cold or distant. Developing the tools to successfully navigate the often difficult waters of a family interaction took some time and came at the cost of some very painful lessons.

One was so painful that it shook me up for days, and reminded me, as no previous case had, that this was not a game, that my customers were very often people going through some of the worst tragedies imaginable, and that every day I had to immerse myself in this "grief soup." I arrived at this particular scene, an apartment on Manhattan's Upper East Side, early one morning, filled with trepidation because the case to which I had been dispatched was the type I always dreaded—a possible SIDS case. Preliminary information on my call-in sheet told me that a newborn had been found unresponsive early that morning and had been pronounced dead at the scene by emergency medical services (EMS).

I walked into an elegant building with a doorman and proceeded upstairs into a fabulous apartment—where I met two parents so consumed with grief and shock that they were almost unresponsive to my greeting. I stepped aside to obtain the story from a detective. It was unremittingly awful. For many years, the parents had tried to conceive a child, and finally with the help of a number of rounds of in vitro fertilization and other therapies, they had been able to birth this baby boy. Because the mother was exhausted by her difficult pregnancy and delivery, the couple decided to hire a baby nurse for their first night home from the hospital.

In the same room with them, also consumed by grief, was the nurse. She told the cops, and me, that some time before dawn she had lain down on the bed in the baby's room, with the infant on her chest; a while later she woke up from a brief nap to find the baby still lying on her chest but gray in color and unresponsive. EMS was unable to resuscitate the child.

I interviewed the nurse for over an hour at the scene, and had her show me precisely how she had been lying on the bed during her nap and how she had positioned the baby. After she did, I immediately suspected that what had happened was a tragic accident. The nurse was a heavyset woman with large, pendulous breasts. She was wearing a thin T-shirt with no bra. From her demonstration, I suspected that during her nap one of her breasts had slipped over the baby's face and smothered him.

For another hour and more, I shuttled back and forth between the nurse in the baby's room and the family in the living room, learning all that I could about the case and at the same time laying the groundwork for a very difficult confrontation. The family was Jewish and was adamant that an autopsy not be performed. From the moment I walked into the apartment, I had known that there was no way this child was going to be buried without having first been autopsied, but I struggled to figure out how I could break the news to the already distraught parents that on top of everything else, I had to take their child away and cut it up. The task was not easy. That morning was one of the most painful of my professional life, but I had to take that child in. While I suspected that the death was accidental, there was no way that OCME or I would permit a dead infant to be buried without first having had a full autopsy to rule out the possibility of foul play.

It took a long time, but finally, with the help of the family's rabbi, I gently convinced the parents that there really was no alternative to the autopsy. I had the baby brought in to the office, and we did the autopsy that day. The case was eventually signed out as an accident, as I suspected it would be, but that was of no comfort to the parents.

A few weeks later, I met with the nurse again, this time at our office. She was accompanied by her boyfriend. I felt as sorry for her as I did for the parents. She was distraught and felt like a murderer. At least I was able to tell her that she would not be indicted for the terrible accidental death of the baby boy. Still later, I was told that she had left the nanny business and the country.

In that terrible case, I had correctly assessed the scene, but in an earlier case, I hadn't—and learned a valuable lesson by my error. My classroom for this lesson was a basement apartment in Harlem. I can still see it now: the cop on duty was outside the building because the apartment was so small that there wasn't room for him to be comfortably inside. He jerked his thumb in the direction of the small kitchen to indicate that was where I'd find the surviving family member.

Entering that kitchen I saw, seated at the table, an older black man, perhaps ninety years old, wearing neat pants and a sweater-vest over a clean but age-yellowed white shirt; a thin man, of quiet dignity, crying silently, tears coursing down his crinkled face. He told me that it was his wife of *seventy* years who had died, and he was very eloquent about how wonderful she was, how much in love they had been. I sat and talked with him for a while, perhaps longer than my job required me to, because in my eyes this man was beautiful.

After a while, I left him sitting in the kitchen and went into the bedroom to examine and photograph the body, and when I pulled back the blanket on the bed, I was stunned: his dead wife was clearly a white woman, of Nordic extraction.

I continued to perform my immediate tasks, which were to take a Polaroid of the deceased woman, and to have the husband sign the Polaroid print and ID form as a positive identification, but I functioned on autopilot. My mind was reeling, trying to imagine the life that this interracial couple must have led in Harlem since the 1920s. In the kitchen, the husband could see the mistake from the look on my face. I had assumed that since the elderly husband sitting in the kitchen was black, his wife must be, and the evidence had proved me wrong. I had even filled out the ID form, while talking with him earlier, inking in her race as black. From his gentle smile as he watched me finish my forms and correct his wife's race, I think he understood that my surprise wasn't at the existence of an interracial couple in Harlem, as there are many such today. He knew that I had assumed, given their age, that she would also be black. He never said a word about my mistake, but I was so embarrassed that I could not summon the courage to ask him about what surely must have been an extraordinary life.

After that vivid lesson on the power of assumption, I strove always to guard against it, attempting to assume nothing when I entered a death scene, so as not to prejudice what I might find. Learning to interact with families, avoid the pitfalls of assumption, and keep my mind open to consideration of all possibilities—these were skills that I could control, abilities that I would come to carry with me into every death scene.

One of the biggest problems that has the potential to disturb a death scene is the human element, which neither the OCME nor an MLI can control. By the time an MLI arrives on a death scene, two or three sets of people have usually been there already: some combination of family-friends-neighbors (who have found the body), the police, and EMS. Although the OCME has primary responsibility for collecting evidence about the death, the presence of these groups on the scene often causes difficulties for us.

On television shows like *CSI,* the viewer watches as the stars arrive at a crime scene to find robust perimeters all set up. No one has disturbed anything. Witnesses sequestered off to the side are ready and eager to spill their guts and all of the resources that the investigators will need to conduct masterful feats of forensic heroics are right at hand.

Real crime scenes aren't so neat.

One of the most difficult tasks that the authorities have to do at a crime scene is preserve its "sanctity" or integrity. Sounds easy, but it's actually quite difficult. In a perfect world, no one other than those directly responsible for investigating the crime would be allowed access to the scene. In reality, protection of the scene is a complicated process, and crime scene perimeters are notoriously leaky.

In New York City, the police usually establish several checkpoints around a homicide scene. There is an outer perimeter (the classic yellow tape we are so familiar with), a handful of intermediate ones, and finally the inner sanctum that is right around the body itself. The duty of guarding these checkpoints usually falls to rookie uniformed officers who may be very effective at keeping out the general public, but who will be hard-pressed to prevent their police bosses from entering. And so generally, at any given homicide, a parade of sightseeing NYPD brass and their acolytes traipse through the scene, usually for no other purpose than to satisfy their curiosity. While professionals such as the crime scene unit and the squad detectives who must try to solve the case have long viewed the permeability of crime scene perimeters as a joke, a basic problem with crime scene contamination begins even *before* the police perimeters are set up.

To be fair, there really is no such thing as a pristine crime scene. The German philosopher Heisenberg's famous observation about the physical universe—that you can't observe something without affecting it—applies in spades to crime scenes. In the real world, crime scenes are, more often then not, very messy places because by the time a perimeter has been set up, all sorts of people have tramped through it—EMS, police officers, the fire department, friends, relatives, neighbors, and even the occasional pizza deliveryman.

At times the contamination of the crime scene by first responders has gotten so bad that EMS came to be referred to around the ME's office as the "Evidence Mangling Service," and its workers, the EMTs, as the "Evidence Mangling Technicians." The service and its workers earned these monikers because of the tendency of EMTs to rush to do CPR and in other ways disturb death scenes even when that is clearly unnecessary. Though many EMTs feel it is their duty to pronounce a person officially deceased, in New York State there is no law requiring a pronouncement ceremony—and in reality, the EMT who lunges toward the body muttering, "I gotta pronounce, I gotta pronounce," often disturbs vital information at the scene. It is quite enough for him to take note of the fatal injuries and indicate the time when the decedent was found.

Regardless of EMT presence, someone is always there before we are because it is only after a person is dead that the ME's office is called. Despite this seemingly logical rule, one memorable "death" scene belied the OCME maxim, "If it ain't dead, don't call us." In this case, we were summoned to an apartment in Brooklyn in which a young woman had apparently killed herself with an overdose of sleeping pills. Emergency medical services had been there, pronounced her very dead, and left the scene. The ME's investigator arrived a few hours later and began to examine the body. Something bothered him, but it took a few moments for him to realize that the body was too warm and relaxed to have been dead for so many hours. He had a stethoscope with him—although it's not part of our usual equipment—and used it to listen to her chest. To his amazement, he could hear a very faint and very slow heartbeat. Emergency medical services was called back to the scene and the woman was rushed to the hospital, where she eventually recovered from her suicide attempt. In classic New York–style chutzpah, after regaining her health, she sued the city because EMS had misdiagnosed her as dead—and won.

Frequently, when we arrive at death scenes, if EMS has been there before us, we find that forensic evidence has been disturbed. Here's why: it all starts with the phone call. If someone finds a relative, a friend, or a neighbor unresponsive, and calls 911, emergency dispatch must send EMS, even if the caller has assured the dispatcher that the person is dead and has died of natural causes. The 911 dispatcher will not take the caller's word for it, and will send the police and EMS just in case there is a chance the unresponsive person might still be alive and could be helped by emergency treatment. In the lingo of 911 operators, these calls are known as "person down," and a person-down designation provokes the highest level of EMS response, a Code Three. So even if the caller describes the body as bloated, smelly, maggot-ridden, and otherwise thoroughly dead, dispatch is still going to send EMS and the police careening to the location with lights flashing and sirens wailing.

Emergency medical technicians do receive a little bit of training on preservation of evidence, but while many EMTs rotate through our office for a few days during their schooling, EMTs in the field often fail to recognize the importance of preserving forensic evidence. To be fair, the duration of the EMT training program is measured in hours, not years, and as a result I've always cut newer EMTs some slack. Veterans, however, should learn from experience how to preserve forensic evidence and a death scene. Much to the detriment of many cases, I've encountered far too many instances of "sightseeing"—EMTs coming into a scene in which the person is long dead, and nevertheless touching this, moving that, and generally acting like tourists. I have been at death scenes where EMTs have walked through pooled blood, disturbed blood splatter, and left their fingerprints on walls—even when the body was obviously decomposed. In the worst example of this interference that I personally encountered, an EMT cut off a bloody shirt to gain access to the body and try to resuscitate the victim, only to put the shirt in a biohazard bag. This particular EMT then went on to throw the shirt away because it had blood on it, an act that destroyed potential evidence.

Despite this bone that I am picking, I have a great deal of respect for EMS and its wonderful medical staff. There is no doubt that quick response and hard work by emergency technicians save lives every day. Most of the police and EMS personnel that I've worked with over the years mean well, and by and large do a great job. Nevertheless, this does not give EMS or anyone else in a position of authority a blank check to hang about a crime scene for no reason, behavior that could be construed as criminal tampering with evidence. Emergency medical technicians are not the only ones who are regularly guilty of this crime. Cops do it, too, mostly rookie patrol officers and neophyte detectives; but I have also been at a death scene in which the chief of detectives decided to go through the pants of a dead man, pants that were hanging over a chair, before I'd had a chance to properly investigate the scene for the ME's office. Since OCME was responsible for making the identification of the bodies, an understanding of proper legal procedure should have mandated that the chief leave things untouched until I'd finished with them.

We MLIs work closely with the men and women of the NYPD, and often with many of the rookies, since one of the traditional jobs given to rookies is "sitting on a DOA," or, in non-cop parlance, waiting with a dead body until the ME's office has arrived and examined and released the body to the family, or until the morgue transportation has arrived and taken the body in for autopsy. We MLIs do our share of teaching these rookies, and not always in the classroom.

The really fresh rookies, just out of the police academy, are easy to spot, as they still display a puppylike eagerness to please. Their uniforms are perfectly creased and starched because they haven't yet been dry-cleaned, and their gun belts are so new that they are shiny and stiff, creaking when the rookies move around. Many of these fine young men and women are clearly nervous around dead bodies, and the more decomposed the body is, the harder it is for me to resist getting them involved. First I tell them—truthfully—that they must remain in the room with me while I examine the body. (This is actual protocol to protect us both in case there are later allegations that valuables are missing from the death scene.) Once I get the rookie into the room, it's awfully hard to resist saying, "Hey, come here and help me turn over this decomp." That's when they usually turn a few shades of green, and bolt. Over the years, I have seen some rookies vomit, and one or two nearly pass out, though most of them just grimly help me while looking like they would rather be anywhere else.

Every so often, I would come across a cop who displayed a surprisingly high level of comfort around dead people. I came to learn that there are quite a number of police officers who have been funeral directors, and even some who continue to moonlight as funeral directors, so when a rookie affected nonchalance at the scene of a spectacularly decomposed body, I was often able to correctly guess why. The NYPD is aware of the value of having cops who are also morticians and knows that they are made-to-order for assignment to the so-called ME squad, an NYPD Missing Persons detective unit permanently attached to OCME.

Though most rookies handle the realities of babysitting a DOA just fine, many find themselves lured in by any of the number of urban legends about cops and dead bodies. With childlike anticipation, the cops would often approach me while at death scenes to ask me about a frequently repeated urban legend concerning a rookie cop and a very dead body. The time is 3:00 A.M., and the rookie is all alone with the corpse, and getting more and more freaked out by that fact, when suddenly, due to rigor mortis, the body bolts upright into a sitting position. The completely terrified cop empties his service revolver into the body, making sure it stays dead.

While many who ask me about this tale would love to believe it, in truth it is nothing more than an urban myth. The key is a misunderstanding of rigor mortis (the literal English translation of the Latin phrase rigor mortis is "the stiffness of death"). It is a biochemical process that brings about the contraction of all the *muscles* of the body after death. Rigor doesn't set in immediately, but rather over a period of hours the contraction process slowly engulfs the entire body until it is rigidly stiff. Rigor mortis generally takes around twelve hours to manifest fully. The stiffness persists for an additional twelve to twenty-four hours, and then dissipates over a further twelve hours, until the body once again becomes floppy.

The mechanism is a chemical one. During life, muscles contract when *actin* and *myosin,* fibers within the muscles, slide together. (The sliding motion of the fibers is akin to what happens when you move your two hands together, interlacing the fingers.) The fibers use calcium ions to form a bond that holds them together. At the same time, the live body is also producing the energy molecule adenosine triphosphate (ATP). The body uses ATP to release the calcium that the fibers have gathered, by knocking the calcium ion out from in between the actin and myosin. This allows the muscle to relax. When a person dies, *actin* and *myosin* fibers continue to grab calcium and slide together, limited only by the availability of intracellular calcium. But since the dead body no longer makes ATP, the fibers cannot release their captured calcium and so the muscles are unable to relax. The result is rigor. Rigor mortis proceeds so slowly, though, that there is not nearly enough oomph in it to make a body sit up; over the course of twelve hours, the body slowly stiffens, freezing in the last position it held.

One question often asked is how rigor mortis eventually dissipates without the production of ATP. The answer lies in the fact that immediately after death, the body starts to decay and this structural deterioration of the muscle fibers slowly causes the calcium bonds to break down. This eventually allows actin and myosin fibers to fall free of one another. High-end steak houses tenderize prime cuts of beef by allowing but controlling this decomposition process, but the chefs more palatably call their process "aging" the beef.

Rigor mortis is just one of many changes occurring naturally in the body after death, changes that are of immense help to homicide investigators. It is through these changes that we can determine many facts at crime scenes, such as when and where a person has died, whether there was a struggle before death, whether the body was moved after death, or even if it has been stored in a freezer for a while.

Unless a body is immediately cremated or embalmed, decomposition commences promptly. There is more to decomp, though, than is generally understood by the lay person. A body usually decomposes in one of two ways, *putrefaction* or *mummification,* though on occasion it decomposes via both pathways simultaneously.

Putrefaction is a very smelly decaying process in which the body is slowly liquefied by autolysis and bacterial activity. Autolysis literally translates as "self-destruction." Here's how it works: Most cells in the human body contain tiny double-walled sacs of powerful digestive enzymes. These sacs, called lysosomes, require ATP to maintain the integrity of their double walls. After death, when the ATP gravy train stops, lysosomes break down, spilling their cargo of acid-like enzymes into the body of the cell. This process is repeated millions and millions of times, all over the body, eventually turning it into mush.

Bacteria also play a key role in the decaying process. Human beings normally harbor well over a hundred types of bacteria and billions of individual organisms, mainly in the digestive tract. In a live, healthy body, the bacteria are mostly kept in balance, but when death stops the working of the immune system that maintained that balance, a dramatic shift occurs. Freed from the drudgery of digesting food *in* the intestinal tract, the bacteria quickly switch to digesting the intestinal tract itself. Soon bacteria spill out of the intestines into the abdominal cavity and begin to attack the organs. They also speed along the body's built-in superhighways, the blood vessels, munching on muscles and skin along the way.

Bacterial digestion of a corpse really puts the putrid in putrefaction. Frenzied microbial feeding produces enormous amounts of gas and fluids, or in other words, bacteria poop. The body swells up and fluids begin to leak out of the various orifices. Putracine, methane, and hydrogen sulfide are examples of the gases that bacteria produce, and some of these stink to high heaven. If you are wondering why these gases are so repulsive to humans, the answer is that evolution has equipped human beings with extremely sensitive noses for the detection of spoiled meat. Those cavemen who were unable to detect that the carcass they were devouring was spoiled died from food poisoning. Those who survived went on to become our ancestors, in part because their olfactory sense allowed them to avoid rotten food and to live long enough to have progeny.

Putrefaction may smell bad to human beings, but it smells like ambrosia to insects and even to some animals. A fly can detect the off-gassing of putrane from a carcass a mile away, in quantities as small as a few parts per billion. Vultures and some scavenging mammals will make a beeline for the source of the aroma that, to them, means dinner.

In the decomposing human body, it is almost a race to see which team can do more damage to the flesh, the bacteria or the lysosomes. No matter which team wins, given a couple of months or so an average human body's soft tissues will completely melt away. Time-lapse photography would show the flesh gradually melting and puddling until all that's left are bones.

The other major pathway of decomposition, *mummification,* usually occurs when something dies in a very hot, dry environment. During the mummification process, moisture evaporates out of the body's soft tissues, which then shrivel up until they have a leatherlike texture and the whole body begins to look like, well, a mummy. The process stops when no further moisture can be wrung from the tissue. Mummies do smell—they have a sort of cheesy/old library book odor—but not nearly as bad as a putrefied body. Most often, when we find a mummified body, putrefaction is absent because both bacteria and enzymes require water to function properly; if the body dries out quickly enough, putrefaction cannot occur. Occasionally we see decomposition simultaneously along both pathways, such as a body whose trunk is putrefied but whose extremities are mummified. This can also happen when one part of the body is exposed to a hot, dry environment and the other exposed to a warm, moist environment, such as happens when a part of a body is wedged against a radiator. The side near the heat source will more likely mummify, while the side exposed to the regular atmosphere in the room will probably putrefy.

Bodies can also mummify if they are freeze-dried. Recently the surprisingly well-preserved body of a World War II aviator was discovered in a northern glacier where the icy environment had mummified it. So perfectly can mummification preserve a body that in R. Dale Guthrie's 1990 book *Frozen Fauna of the Mammoth Steppe,* the professor emeritus at the University of Alaska describes several colleagues' and his experience dining on a stew made from the meat of "Blue Babe," a 36,000-year-old bison carcass that had been found frozen in the tundra. Guthrie wrote of the experience, "The meat was well aged but still a little tough," while another of the diners described the meal as "agreeable."

When a once-frozen body—whether a human corpse or a frozen piece of meat from an ordinary kitchen refrigerator—thaws, it decomposes much faster then a body that was never frozen. This happens because ice crystals form inside the cells during freezing and the crystals disrupt the integrity of cell walls, making it easier for putrefaction to occur.

Mostly though, when people think of mummies, it's not the icy kind that they picture. Rather they think of the Mediterranean variety that inhabit Hollywood films—linen-wrapped monsters who rush about trying to eat living people. Let me assure you that nothing is less likely to attack a human being than a dead body, particularly one that's been dead and buried in a pyramid for three thousand years. As for that, the ancient Egyptians' secret for making their dead into mummies was not wrapping the bodies in linen, or pulling the brain out of the nose with a long metal hook. Nor was it stuffing the abdominal cavity with flowers and garlic, though the evisceration was helpful to mummification because it prevented putrefaction. The secret lay in Egypt's geography, which then as now abutted an enormous desert featuring almost zero humidity and temperatures that can climb above 120 degrees Fahrenheit. Anthropologists speculate that early Egyptians, traveling through the desert, came across the bodies of animals that had died and had naturally mummified in the extreme environment. Obsessed with the afterlife, these travelers would have been fascinated by the relatively lifelike appearance of a dead animal that had been preserved by mummification. It is easy to imagine those early embalmers—for that is essentially what they were—experimenting with this preservation technique and incorporating it into their religious practice.

Whichever path you travel on, be it putrefaction or mummification, the ultimate destination for all of us is the same: ashes to ashes, dust to dust; like it or not, we all rot.

FIVE

ON COUNTLESS TELEVISION crime shows and in just as many crime novels, the pop-up ME magically appears at every crime scene, does a cursory examination, and immediately tells the hero/detective, "This guy died at 11:27 yesterday morning."

Sorry, wrong number—way too precise!

One of the most basic tasks for an MLI at a death scene is pinning down the approximate time of death. The first step in doing so is to establish the "postmortem interval" (PMI). This is the range of time between when the person was last absolutely known to be alive and when the person was found dead. Thus the PMI is not a fancy way of saying "how long has this person been dead?" but a device that we use to identify a clear window of time during which the decedent must have changed from being alive to being dead. Despite what television crime dramas would have you believe about "time of death," it is often impossible to discern the exact moment during the PMI when someone expired. And because a mistake can have such grave consequences, I am always careful when giving a time of death to let families or detectives know that what I am providing them with is "approximate." Too many cops, as well as too many families of victims, have seen too many TV crime shows.

Establishing the PMI and an approximate time of death is absolutely critical if the death is suspected of being anything other than from natural causes. In a homicide, if we can determine that interval with good accuracy, the police can then question suspects as to their whereabouts at the presumed time of death. If a suspect can't provide a good alibi, then there is strong circumstantial evidence that he or she is connected to the crime.

Here are the facts about what it is possible for us to do in regard to estimating the time of death within the PMI. In the first twenty-four hours after a body is dead, we are pretty good at pinpointing the time, and can do it generally within a four-hour block. If the body has been dead less than twelve hours, we can do even better, coming up with as little as a two-hour block in which the death occurred. However, once the body has been dead longer than twenty-four hours, the task becomes more difficult. If the body has lain undetected from between twenty-four and forty-eight hours, we'll be able to locate the time of death within a six- to eight-hour block. If it has been dead for forty-eight to seventy-two hours, which is three days, we can usually offer the detectives a twelve-hour block as the approximate time of death. But beyond seventy-two hours? Frankly, if the body has lain undetected for more than three days, we'll be guessing in twenty-four-hour blocks when we approximate the time of death.

Attempting to fix a position in *time* is not really all that different from attempting to fix a physical location in *space*. The more points of reference you can gather about the location you are attempting to verify, the greater your accuracy will be. That's why cross streets are so helpful when getting driving directions, and why navigators on ships of old used a sextant to "shoot" the position of three stars, which allowed them to more exactly locate their longitude and latitude. Similarly, locating an unknown particular point in time, such as when a person died, requires using as many indicators as possible to narrow the interval and produce the safest guess possible.

We start by using three early postmortem changes, one of which, *rigor mortis,* I've already described. The other two are *algor mortis* (temperature of death) and *livor mortis* (color of death). Each of these three changes develops in a dead body along a well-documented timeline that we can utilize in determining the time of death in some cases.

Rigor mortis's timeline is one of the first things taught to MLIs. As I described earlier, it takes about twelve hours after death for a body to reach full rigor; then full rigor persists from twelve to twenty-four hours after which point the body enters the third period as rigor gradually relaxes over the next twelve hours. Part of becoming an experienced MLI is learning how to recognize which phase of rigor a body might be in. We learn how to determine if the decedent is going into or coming out of rigor. One variable you always have to take into account at a scene, in this regard, is the ambient environment. Rigor is biochemical, and like all such processes, it is subject to temperature fluctuations. Very cold temperatures will slow down the onset of rigor, while exposure to heat or even great physical exertion before death will accelerate its arrival. At first, it's not so easy to figure out where exactly in the timeline a body might be, but the ability to make a better-educated guess can be learned; one way to raise the level of your guess is to combine rigor clues with clues from algor and livor.

Algor mortis, or the "temperature of death," is also a good measure of time passing. The first step in obtaining this information is to ascertain the core temperature, or the body's inner temperature. Another urban legend has it that the ME punches a hole in the body with a meat-locker thermometer, piercing the liver in order to take that temperature—and in the process, leaving a big hole for the mortician to repair. This is one legend that has a basis in fact. While there used to be a practice of going for the liver, this is no longer considered necessary. Today we use a good, old-fashioned, albeit a rather long rectal thermometer to obtain the core temperature, which works just as well—even though the use of such a thermometer usually raises some eyebrows among the rookie cops.

After a while, I had the routine down pat and rather enjoyed the cop's predictable discomfort. I would do it slowly and right in front of the rookie so that he or she could follow my every move. I'd take out a condom and roll it down over a rectal thermometer before inserting that thermometer into the decedent's anus. The explanation for employing the condom, of course, is that we do plan to reuse such thermometers, and the condom keeps them clean. We do dispose of the used condoms after a single use.

Once obtained, the core temperature also helps us to estimate the time of death within the PMI. After the first few hours following death, the dead body loses a degree to a degree-and-a-half per hour, until it reaches equilibrium with its surroundings. So if the ambient temperature (the temperature in the room where the body is lying) is 70 degrees and the core body temperature has dropped from 98.6 degrees to 70 degrees, we are able to figure that the person has been dead at least 28 hours.

Here again, environmental factors play a role, and you must always be on guard not to glibly state an approximate time of death without taking those factors into consideration. A body will lose its warmth much quicker in very cold places—a homicide victim stuffed into a freezer—than a body lying on a hot roof baking under a summer sun. I was once called to a scene of a young woman who was sunbathing at "Tar Beach," which is what New Yorkers call their roofs during the summer. Sunbathing alone, she had gotten drunk on margaritas while lying on a canvas lounger. She was found dead late in the afternoon by a neighbor, and when I arrived and took her temperature, it was 110 degrees Fahrenheit. Here temperature helped us understand the cause of death but was not much use in establishing the approximate time of death.

A third clue to the time of death derives from the livor mortis, or the lividity of the body. Lividity means the "color" of death, and the color in question derives from pooling blood. During life, most of a person's blood supply inhabits the capillary portion of the circulatory system. Capillaries are the network of tiny vessels that connect your arteries to your veins. After death, with the heart no longer pumping, the blood, subject to gravity, begins to pool in the capillaries instead of flowing through them. Capillaries are very thin walled—only one cell thick. So, very quickly, the pooling blood becomes heavier than the capillary walls can bear, and the walls rupture, spilling blood into the surrounding tissues.

As with rigor and algor mortis, lividity also progresses in predictable fashion. It is always found along the bottom or "dependent" part of the body (whichever side is touching the ground or nearest to the ground), because that is where gravity will pull the blood. Early on, in a light-skinned person, lividity appears pink and lacy, as the first wisps of blood escape into the tissues and begin to stain the skin. As time passes, the pooling blood will turn the skin darker and darker, from pink to red, to purple, and finally to black.

Another way of determining early lividity from more advanced staining is to try the "blanch" test. Early lividity is "blanchable," while very developed lividity will be "fixed," meaning that it has permanently stained the tissues.

If a living person pinches his or her own fingertip firmly for five seconds, then lets it go quickly, the color will change. During the pinching, it will blanch, or whiten, because the pressure pushes the blood out and away from the site of the pinch, leaving that part white. But when the pinch is released, the blood returns and colors the finger once again. On a living person, the blood returns because the heart pumps it back. With a dead body, if we press on an early-livid area, it blanches for a moment but then recolors as gravity pulls the blood back. If we pinch or press a site on the body where blood has pooled, and that site no longer blanches, we know the lividity is fixed, more developed. Lividity usually becomes fixed sixteen hours or so after death.

Further clues to the time of death come from such signs as the degree of clouding in the cornea, from the skin over the abdomen turning a certain greenish color, and from what we call the "drying artifact," the drying of fingers, toes, lips, tongue, and sclera.

These clues are just a few that the *body* can yield. Death scenes offer many more tidbits that can help an MLI pin down just when the body he or she is examining ceased to function. Mail and newspaper delivery, for example, are important items to check. If a person was in the habit of picking up his mail every day, knowing which day he stopped is helpful. How many days of newspapers are piled up outside the front door? That can be a clue as to when the person stopped going out.

But the mother of all important questions to ask before an MLI does or says anything at a scene regarding time of death is, *"Does anyone know the last time this person was seen alive?"* Many times, asking that one simple question spared me embarrassment. Which means, of course, that *until* I learned to ask it—in my first year or so of work—

I called more than one detective back to readjust my time-of-death estimate.

It's not only rookie cops who can get freaked out by a corpse. While I understood from my training that rigor mortis could not make a dead body suddenly sit up, I have to admit I was entirely unprepared for the sounds that a dead body produces.

The first time I heard a body groan, the hair stood up on my arms and the back of my neck, and I froze, until I realized what the source must be: a build-up of gas bubbles produced in the course of decomposition. As the bubbles leak out of the lungs, stomach, and rectum, they make dead bodies groan, burp, and fart—sounds that are sometimes also generated when the body is moved.

I quickly became accustomed to listening to dead people sounding off. But there was another thing I regularly ran into at the scene that I never got used to. It gave me shivers up and down my spine up until my final day at OCME. Every MLI has their "thing," the uncontrollable fear they dread coming across at death scenes. For some investigators, it's rats; for others, maggots. Now I never really had a problem with maggots (okay, maybe a little on my first day), and rats are kinda cute, like squirrels without the bushy tails. For me it was something else. And of course the most awful sight that I ever encountered at a scene involved my nemesis.

The scene: Chinatown. Top floor of a five-story walk-up. In the kitchen, lying on the floor, the mummified body of an elderly, ninety-pound Chinese woman who is long dead. Enter the boyish-looking MLI. I turn her over and it happens—hundreds of *cockroaches* come pouring out of her mouth, like something out of *Freak Show.* Today, if I close my eyes, I can still conjure up the details of the sight. I was up on that kitchen table so fast that I broke the Olympic record for the Jewish high jump.

But as much as I hated roaches, I learned that they and many other insects and their activity are helpful to an MLI in determining the PMI. Because some flies can detect a rotting carcass from a mile away, they maneuver to the putrefying flesh with one goal in mind: laying their eggs. Once flies have laid their eggs in the flesh and those eggs become larva, they are known as maggots. Maggots are anatomically strange creatures: Their nose is in their rear end, alongside their butt. Perhaps this is because they spend most of the day facedown in rotting flesh. From the larval stage, they then reach the pupal stage, the cocoon, which hatches the mature fly. The length of time that it takes for each stage to develop is known and helps us calculate how long a body has been lying dead. Another clue is in the number of stages that we can count on the body. If, for example, it displays pupae as well as maggots, then we know that the body has lain there for more than one full insect-growth cycle.

Despite the emphasis placed on the ME determining the time of death on television shows and in novels, in reality PMI/time of death is just one of many conclusions along with cause and manner of death and verifying the identity of the deceased that we need to make in a scene investigation. Each MLI has his or her own style of investigating. In terms of the PMI, I developed a style of working backward, from the last known moment that the decedent was seen alive, forward, to the moment when the body was found. To perform that calculation, and to determine the cause and manner of death, I have to first relate the body to the scene. Is the position of the body "sensible"? By sensible I mean, does its placement make sense. If, for example, the body is fully clothed, does it make sense for the body to be lying peacefully on the bed? That could mean the body has been moved; but not necessarily. It could also mean, conversely, that the person got dressed, then felt ill, and lay down without undressing again. We find many bodies in bathrooms, kitchens, back halls, even inside closets. I discovered one man hunched over in the bottom of his clothes closet; perhaps he had gone there, in the throes of his final illness, because that was where he felt safest.

And I can't count the number of dead bodies that I have pulled off toilets. I learned that bodies found on toilets were usually there taking a "terminal crap." The explanation of the term is, again, logical: when you're attempting to evacuate your bowel, you push, you bear down, and this process lowers your heart rate. This happens because by bearing down you increase the pressure in your chest and squeeze the vagus nerve, which is a major player of the parasympathetic nervous system. While the sympathetic nervous system acts in the body like a gas pedal in a car, the parasympathetic acts like a brake. Hitting the brake can throw the body into a terminal bradycardia, meaning that the heart slows down to the point where it can stop. Thus the phrase: terminal crap. You bear down, your heart slows and stops, and you die on the bowl. Avoiding this ignominious end might be best done by following my grandmother's Old World recipe for a long life: eat four stewed prunes a day, and don't push too hard.

Similarly, there is a misconception that when you die, you lose control of your anal sphincter and defecate in your pants. Not so. To defecate requires contraction pressure of pelvic muscles and contraction of the smooth muscle in the rectum. You don't defecate if those muscles are relaxed by death. If there is fecal matter in the very end of the rectum, some might leak out of a relaxed anal sphincter when the body is moved, but there will be no full-fledged active pooping once the body is dead. A related urban legend is that after death, hair and the fingernails of the body continue to grow. This has become a staple of horror movies where the corpse has more hair in death than it did in life, and has fingernails that in the coffin have become like claws. Not true. Death stops the processes of growth in hair, teeth, and fingernails. What does happen, though, is drying. The skin of the fingers dries, and in the drying process, the skin appears to recede, thus revealing more of the underlying nail than you would see on a finger in life. The same is true with the scalp.

After establishing the body's relationship to the scene, I survey the surroundings. Are they in order or disarray? If there is disorder, is it the sort that would have been made by a usually sloppy person, or by an intruder or some other disturber of the scene? Are there signs of a struggle or a robbery? I look into the medicine cabinet, the garbage, and the refrigerator for clues as to what might have caused the death. What has the decedent been eating lately? Are the medicine bottles on the cabinet shelf, or out on the counter—the latter possibly indicating more frequent or more recent use?

Only after I have examined the context of the dead body in its surroundings—and taken many photographs of those surroundings—do I take photos of the body itself, and then I begin to investigate it.

I always have to disrobe the body, because clothing can conceal damage. Once, a body was found sitting, fully clothed, and without external signs of violence, in the waiting room of a city hospital. When we disrobed the body, we found a bullet hole under the arm, high up in the armpit. The man had been shot to death, the bloody clothes removed, the body cleansed of external blood, then reclothed, and taken to the hospital's emergency waiting room, where—the murderer or his assistants correctly figured—it could sit in a chair for a long time without being noticed, certainly for long enough to permit them to make their escape.

As I spent more time at the OCME, I learned more about matters that had been in the headlines in recent years, but that I had not paid much attention to prior to joining the office. While I had known that Dr. Hirsch's appointment was relatively recent, I came to learn the history that led to his appointment as chief medical examiner (CME). This had occurred in 1989, after Mayor Edward Koch fired the previous CME, Dr. Elliot Gross, who had been appointed by Koch in 1979 following the dismissal of Dr. Gross's predecessor, Dr. Michael Baden.

According to published reports, both Dr. Baden and Dr. Gross were considered highly competent pathologists, but deficient as managers of the country's largest ME's office. Dr. Baden's dismissal came after Mayor Koch received negative reports on Dr. Baden's administering of the OCME from the city's health commissioner and from the Manhattan DA. These officials contended that Dr. Baden had lost important evidence in homicide cases and had been unresponsive to requests from their respective offices. In turn, Dr. Baden sued the city for wrongful dismissal, and that suit wound its way through the courts until it was rejected by a federal appeals court in 1986. Dr. Gross, who took over the office following Baden's departure, was also fired by Koch; his termination came after charges—later dismissed—of professional misconduct.

Dr. Hirsch's advent to the office was more than changing the chief executive. The city chose Dr. Charles Hirsch to rescue the beleaguered agency and restore that agency's tarnished reputation. New York could not have made a better choice, because Dr. Hirsch brought with him a whole new philosophy on how death investigations should be conducted and who should conduct them. Before the Hirsch era, death investigations for the ME's office had been done mostly by freelancers, doctors who were per diem contractors. These physicians practiced in various fields of clinical medicine ranging from general practice to urology, but by and large had little or no formal training in forensics. They went about their days seeing live patients, making rounds at hospitals, even performing surgery, all the while carrying beepers provided by the ME's office. When a death was reported to OCME, the communications unit would start paging the doctor who was listed as on duty. It was often hours before the "tour doctor," as he or she was known, would respond to the communications unit, and often many more hours before the doctor would investigate the case. One of my fellow MLIs, who before becoming a PA had been a New York City cop for twenty-one years, told me that in the late 1960s during his rookie year he was assigned to sit on a DOA for his four-to-twelve shift. He was relieved at midnight with still no sign of the ME. After his return to work the next day, he was reassigned to the same DOA, still waiting for the ME to arrive.

Even when OCME tour doctors did deign to show up, some of these freelancers did "drive-by" investigations, cursory at best. Occasionally, they did not even bother visiting the death scene in person but simply telephoned the police on duty there, asked them a few questions, noted down the cops' observations and conclusions, and wrote them up as the OCME's conclusions, as though they had actually been at the scene.

When Dr. Hirsch arrived on the scene in 1989, his administration inherited the old investigators, and, as typically happens in city bureaucracy, he could not simply dismiss those tour doctors that he felt were not performing up to his standards. Determined to purge the agency of the worst of them, he dutifully followed the city's arcane labor rules, and at that pace, it took almost a decade to get rid of them all. During that time, at least one tour doctor was indicted on charges of submitting fraudulent travel expense sheets for death scenes that he never actually visited.

I must point out that some of the tour doctors did splendid work, and there are still three of the per diem doctors working for OCME in our Staten Island office, where they are well regarded. However, even before he arrived in New York City, Dr. Hirsch had determined to replace the part-time tour doctor system of investigation with investigators who were better trained for the specific task of death investigations—and he had just the model in mind. When he had earlier come to Suffolk County, New York, from Cleveland, Ohio, he had inherited the country's first MLI corps composed exclusively of PAs, a program established by his Suffolk County predecessor. Part of Dr. Hirsch's attractiveness to Mayor Koch was his intent to begin a similar MLI corps to deal with the much larger jurisdiction of the city of New York. These investigators would be properly trained in death investigation, and would be available twenty-four hours a day, and they would not have private practices that could distract them from their postmortem duties. With a corps of *full-time* MLIs, no excuses would be tolerated for the ME's office not responding quickly to death scenes. The corps was designed and trained to perform death investigation better, more professionally, and more thoroughly than had ever been done before in New York. Shortly after Dr. Hirsch arrived in New York, he publicly stated that he was staking his professional reputation on the success of the new corps of investigators. We new recruits were imbued with this spirit of reform, on being part of a new administration that was going to turn death investigation in the Big Apple on its head.

Once the MLI corps program got started in New York City, there *were* dramatic changes in the way the ME's office went about its work, and if the general public never noticed, professionals such as the cops certainly did. Evidence that there was, indeed, a new sheriff in town came in such statistics as our response time; the average time it took us to respond to a death scene dropped from a lethargic half a day to a prompt within the hour. Precinct detectives, accustomed to many years of legendary poor response from the ME's office, were shocked to receive calls from uniformed officers at scenes, saying, "Get over here now, the ME's here." And when the detectives did arrive at the scene, and encountered one of the new MLIs, they soon realized that we were very good at what we did. We took our work seriously, and in turn expected to be treated with respect by our law enforcement colleagues. Even so, it was about three years into the MLI program before there was widespread acceptance by the detectives of our presence—and our competence—at death scenes.

Even after the MLI corps as a whole were accepted by our police colleagues, rookie MLIs still had to make their own reputations out on the street if they expected to be taken seriously. When I arrived at OCME, it was explained to me that there were three levels of MLIs—or rather there were supposed to be three levels: I, II, and III. In practice, though, there were only two levels: I and II. On Level I, you were supervised. On Level II, you were able to handle cases entirely on your own without a supervisor present or even checking your work when you returned to the office. As a young MLI-II, I gloried in the responsibility and lack of someone looking over my shoulder; but looking back, I realize that my colleagues and I would probably have benefited from some closer supervision. But in typical bureaucratic fashion, the city did not get around to creating the MLI-III position until 2005, sixteen years after Dr. Hirsch took office. Prior to its formalization, an in-office title of Senior MLI was used to designate those MLIs who demonstrated leadership qualities and excellent investigative skills.

About ten months after I began at OCME, there came a moment when I was working with a body in an apartment, holding its arms with mine as I turned it over, peering into its eyes for signs of disease and what not, and doing it all so smoothly and correctly that my supervisor said to me, "Now you're dancing." In that instant, I got the overwhelming sensation that I was finally coming to understand what was expected of me as an investigator. I was almost there, almost ready to move up to Level II.

A few weeks and perhaps a hundred death scenes later, the supervisor stayed in the car as I walked up to the sixth floor in a Lower East

Side tenement building to examine a dead person and speak with his family. It was not the first time the supervisor had stayed in the car while I worked, but I sensed it could be the last.

The moment is vivid in my mind. I remember a whitewashed brick building with narrow stairs on which the linoleum was so worn with use that the steps themselves seemed indented; in my mind's eye, I can see my brown work shoes on those stairs—skipping down the stairs, exhilarated, because I knew, just knew, that I had handled everything upstairs perfectly and hadn't at any point felt the need to call down to the car to ask for guidance.

The scene upstairs had been chaotic with what I would come to dub the "noisy quiet," the unsettled and far-from-silent chaos of a death scene, filled with milling police, a distraught and grieving family, and a body that needed examination. During my time in that apartment—less than an hour—I had not only been able to "dance" properly with the body but also to perform another necessary task: to answer the family's questions, and to interview and soothe them. At the same time, I was able to speak on the phone with the funeral director and make sure that the family understood the next steps in the process. In that apartment, I had been the subject matter expert, and had not only done my job but also certified to myself that I was ready to go on to the next level of medicolegal investigation, to become an MLI-II. I would no longer need to rely on supervision. From here on out, I would be on my own.

SIX

BEING AN MLI-II means that you're a seasoned pro, but it also means that the responsibility for every case falls squarely on your shoulders. Sometimes that means listening to what the cops have to say; sometimes that means solving the cops' case for them.

One day I was called to a bloody scene in a Harlem apartment and was greeted at the door by two impatient detectives from the local precinct—impatient because they could not touch the body until I got there, and they had been waiting for me quite a while. Cops sitting and waiting for the MLI to arrive and do his job is the usual state of affairs when a death scene is presumed to be a homicide scene—but you would not know that from the depictions of homicide investigations in most television crime shows.

Your average television crime show generally highlights the exploits of a few cops, the same ones in every episode, cops who seem to catch every interesting case in the city. The detective stars always arrive at crime scenes to find the Crime Scene Unit (CSU) and the ME already there, finished with their work, and each having prepared a short speech from which our heroes will glean all the clues they need. Straying even further from reality, the ME usually appears on screen more for effect than for substance because often the television detectives don gloves and examine the body themselves. Then, armed with the results of a perfect crime scene investigation, our intrepid stars go out and follow every lead by themselves until they solve the crime. What's more, they do all this in sixty minutes—less the time for commercials.

Reality is messier, slower, and less dependent on star detectives. Major crimes, especially homicides, are not solved by lone detectives egged on by their incredibly savvy and perpetually irritated bosses. Complex crimes are solved by teamwork. There are about 40,000 cops in the NYPD, including more than 3,000 detectives. Every borough has at least two specialized homicide detective units, but, unlike what happens in television shows, the detectives in the homicide units are never the primary investigators of a case. The detectives in the homicide unit merely supplement the work of the *precinct* detectives who actually catch the case.

When 911 is called to report that a body has been found, the 911 operator relays the call to an RMP (an archaic term standing for radio-mounted patrol car) covering that sector of the local precinct. The RMP's uniformed officers respond to the call; and unless the perp (perpetrator) was stupid enough to have hung around, the uniforms' primary job is to secure the crime/death scene. If this is an obvious homicide, or a possible one, a patrol supervisor will also respond, and often so will the precinct commander. While they are doing so, the precinct's desk sergeant will notify the precinct's detective squad.

Once the commanding officer of that detective squad (usually a detective lieutenant) has been notified of a DOA, he will dispatch two detectives to the scene. The squad commander will also pass the information on to the borough's homicide squad commander, who will send over a detective or two to help out. The homicide detectives will remain attached to the local precinct for at least the first seventy-two hours of the ensuing investigation.

This is done because the first three days of a homicide investigation are critical, since most of the cases that do get solved are cracked from clues picked up in this time period. Because of inaccurate portrayals of police work on television, most people are unaware that the precinct detectives have primary responsibility at homicide scenes. Homicide squad detectives function as temporary labor, augmenting the manpower of the local precinct during the early days of an investigation.

Next, the squad commander will alert another specialized unit of detectives, the CSU. In New York City, CSU is based in the Police Crime Lab in Queens, and from there responds to every major crime in the five boroughs. And even with lights and sirens, they often get bottled up in traffic.

Just as no one is supposed to touch a body until the ME arrives, so too no one is to enter a homicide scene or examine the body until CSU has finished its work. To do otherwise is to risk the destruction of valuable forensic evidence and invite withering cross-examination from defense attorneys who will want an explanation as to why proper crime scene protocol was not followed.

New York Police Department's CSU usually requires at least a couple of hours to process a scene because a surprising amount of work is involved. First they must photograph the scene and the body, then measure all the dimensions of the crime scene and create a sketch of it, indicating on the drawing the position and location of the body and of any other evidence they might have noticed. Then they dust for fingerprints, and finally they collect evidence such as weapons, shell casings, spent rounds, drugs, drug paraphernalia, and so on. Only when all of this has been accomplished can the body be examined by the MLI.

After CSU has been contacted, the precinct desk sergeant also makes a number of other phone calls to various police brass and to the assistant DA on duty. Eventually the sergeant will notify the ME's office, but often not until an hour or two after the case has first been reported. The result is that the ME invariably arrives at the scene well *after* the detectives.

So when I arrived at that reported homicide scene in Harlem, I was not surprised to be met at the door by impatient detectives, who I knew were not upset with me. A great deal goes into processing a crime scene, and it wasn't my "tardiness" that was holding things up or causing their anxiety. Even if I had arrived earlier, the detectives would have had to wait, along with me, since CSU was not nearly finished with their work. The waiting was par for the course; in all the years that I performed scene investigations for the ME's office, I recall only a very few cases where I arrived at a homicide scene *after* CSU was done.

Hanging around and drinking endless cups of coffee with the cops, just outside the scene, as we waited and the body stiffened, was *de rigeur.*

On this occasion, when I stuck my head in the apartment door shortly after I arrived, the lead CSU detective told me he still had about an hour to go, so while waiting I chatted with the precinct detectives and got "the story." They told me that the decedent, who was lying on his back on the floor in a pool of blood, had been a member of a band that had been using the apartment to rehearse. They said he had died of gunshot wounds, and that they already had a prime suspect in custody, the band's lead singer, whom they had taken in for questioning at the "house," the local precinct. However, the suspect wasn't singing a tune that the cops were buying; instead, he was claiming self-defense—that there had been a scuffle, and the gun had gone off accidentally. Since no one else had been in the room at that moment except the shooter and the dead man, it might prove difficult for the police to refute the suspect's song.

By the time CSU finished and invited me in, I had donned the white Tyvec overalls, hood, and booties that we wear at every homicide scene so as not to track in new evidence. I ducked under the yellow tape stretched across the apartment door and entered the scene. The decedent lay supine on the floor of a rear bedroom. A brief survey of the scene and a first glance at the body seemed to support the cops' belief that two shots had been fired—there were two holes in a wall of the bedroom, and the decedent had two apparent gunshot wounds. The large pool of blood underneath him seemed also to buttress their belief that one shot had gone through his chest, out his back, and then into the wall, and that the second had grazed the victim's head as he went down, and then also had gone on to hit the wall. When I examined the decedent, though, I found something that the detectives and CSU had not seen.

But I wasn't quite ready to delve into it, yet. First I had to figure out the approximate time of death. Neighbors had told detectives of hearing an altercation earlier in the day and of loud popping sounds from the apartment. I began my examination of the body by ascertaining the state of the decedent's *rigor, livor,* and *algor mortis,* which verified a decedent time of death consistent with the neighbors' recollections.

Then I turned my attention to his wounds. I quickly confirmed that the head wound was superficial and would not have killed him. A shallow graze over his right temple, it had torn through the skin on an upward angle; this led me to suspect that the decedent had been ducking or falling at the time that bullet struck. Next were the torso wounds. There were two, one in the chest and the other was where I suspected it would be, in his back.

Thus far, all evidence continued to support the initial assessment of two shots, both hitting the victim and then the wall. But I had learned the hard way, over the years, not to judge too quickly, and so I continued my examination.

Before inspecting the chest wound itself, I looked at the surrounding skin and clothing, searching carefully for signs of fouling (soot) or stippling (embers). The presence of one or both of these types of gunpowder residue would indicate that this had been a close or contact gunshot. While there had been no such deposits on the victim's head, I found a small amount of stippling on the front of the decedent's button-up shirt, around the hole the bullet had made as it entered the victim's chest—but I found no fouling.

Fouling is the name given to the ash produced from completely burned gunpowder, ash that settles on the skin or clothing around an entrance wound, but only does so when the muzzle of the gun is less than one foot from the victim. Very lightweight, the ash cannot travel in the air more than a foot or so without being dispersed. Moreover, once it settles onto a surface, it can be easily disturbed, and an investigator must take care not to accidentally wipe off this often vital evidence. *Stippling* is a term describing dark little pinpoint burns that look like black pepper and surround a wound if the muzzle flash of the gun was within three feet of the victim. Stippling occurs because small chunks of burning gunpowder follow the bullet out of the gun as though they were tiny satellite bullets, and embed themselves into the skin or clothes of the victim. Unlike fouling, which drifts like a cloud, the heavier embers that cause stippling travel at great speed, for up to three feet from the gun, and once embedded on a surface are much more difficult to remove.

The presence of stippling on the decedent's shirt, combined with the absence of fouling meant that the muzzle of the gun had been between one and three feet away from the victim at the time that shot was fired. Things were getting interesting.

Now I could finally examine the torso wounds. The first thing to establish was precisely where the bullet had entered and exited. It was a no-brainer that the hole in the decedent's chest was the entrance wound, since it was surrounded by stippling. But even had the stippling not been present, I could have deduced that the hole in the chest was the entrance wound because its margin was defined by a characteristic abrasion ring that hallmarks an entrance wound. When a bullet enters flesh, the skin around the entrance spot is "shored," that is, the underlying tissue braces the skin so that, as the bullet drags the skin into the underlying tissue, it produces a rim of bruising around the entrance spot. An exit wound usually appears different: since there is no underlying tissue layer to similarly cushion the skin, the bullet exits by stretching the skin until it tears through. The resultant wound is usually slitlike and has no bruised margins.

But when I turned over the dead musician, I found that the wound in his back looked almost identical to the entrance wound in front. This back wound also had the classic abrasion ring. After pondering this for a moment, I had a hunch. Using my gloved hand to push aside the pooled and partially coagulated blood under the victim, I found in the parquet floor beneath his body, a tiny pockmark, so small that if I hadn't been looking for it, it might have escaped detection. Eureka! The wound on the decedent's back was indeed an exit wound, but a very special type—a *shored* exit.

The unusual exit wound and the slug that would later be dug out of the floor underneath the pockmark (the bullet from a *third* shot) established something very important to the investigation: The victim had been *shot while lying on the floor.* How did I know? Because as this third bullet exited, the floor had braced the skin on the decedent's back, and the skin was dragged into the floor, causing damage identical to that of an entrance wound.

Now I was ready to reassess the scene. Fortified with the knowledge that three shots had been fired, I was able to reconstruct the likely sequence of events. The first shot had been taken from more than three feet away from the victim. It had grazed the decedent in his head, knocking him down, and then buried itself in the wall. The shooter then fired the second shot, also from some distance away, a shot that missed the falling victim entirely and also ended up lodged in the wall. I knew those first two shots *had* to have been fired from at least three feet or more away because they left no powder burns on the victim. Another clue to the distance was that the second shot missed completely. Even a five-year-old would have been able to hit a grown man from a distance of three feet. After the first two shots, the shooter had strolled closer to his victim who was by then lying helpless on the floor, dazed, possibly unconscious from the head wound, and he fired the third and final bullet into his victim's chest—a fatal shot in more ways then one since it left the clue that would prove to be the shooter's undoing.

With a new understanding of the sequence of events in hand, including that there had been three shots, the cops put their suspect in the "box" at the station house and told him a white lie. They said he had missed a witness who had been hiding in a closet at the time of the shooting. The cops reconstructed the murder scene for the suspect: "You came in; the two of you had an argument; there was a scuffle; your first shots knocked him down, and then, while he was on the floor, you fired into his chest, killing him."

It was the detail of the singer having shot his victim while on the floor that pushed the suspect to believe the police did have a witness who could later testify against him in court. In reaction, he confessed to the murder then and there, in the hope of obtaining a better plea deal from the prosecutors.

This "trouble in the band" case occurred during the early 1990s, a time when there were many murders in New York City, and cops, EMS, and OCME personnel considered Harlem to be homicide central. On another sweltering hot July morning, I was called to a homicide scene in a Harlem housing project. Housing projects in New York City were dismal and sad places; at night they could be downright scary. We MLIs hated being called to housing project death scenes because invariably the body would be on the top floor and the elevator would not be functioning.

If a Harlem housing project call came in at night, often we would not go directly to the scene, but instead to the local precinct and pick up a police officer to escort us to the body. Yes, there was a cop sitting with the DOA waiting for us. But getting up to where the body was sometimes meant traveling through some of the roughest turf in the city's crack wars, which at the time was the major source of the city's homicide problem. Desk sergeants at precincts would not dole out cops for such escort duty without exacting their pound of flesh. Whenever I'd walk into a precinct at 2:00 A.M. and ask for an escort to a death scene, the sergeant would always produce the smallest female officer on duty, and say, "Officer, will you please escort this much-larger-than-you *man* to the DOA?" I took their ribbing and kept a smile on my face, because if I was going to walk up fifteen flights of very scary, poorly lit housing project stairs at 2:00 A.M., I wanted to be walking behind anyone who had a gun.

That morning the case to which I was called required no escort because the victim was found during daylight hours, in a ground-floor stairwell. He seemed very young to me, with a face not yet ready to shave, maybe fifteen or sixteen. He had several bullet holes in him, two condoms in his back pocket, and a scattering of crack cocaine vials lay on the floor around him. On this particular day, I was being trailed by two PA students who were rotating through our office from somewhere in the Midwest, and also by a roving reporter for *Advance,* a monthly magazine for PAs. Because the initial report was sent out over police radios as a double homicide (the other victim had been taken to a nearby hospital in hopes of saving her, which the hospital personnel were unable to do), television crews had also responded and were waiting outside the building. Also present were the usual thirty to forty police personnel who tend to swarm at crime scene like this one; and of course, this being New York City, a large and boisterous crowd had gathered, easily three hundred strong.

It was a bloody scene inside that stairwell, and there was not much room to move around, so by the time I finished examining the victim, I had gotten some of his blood on the sleeves of my shirt. I exited the building and headed toward the police CSU van where I knew I could find a hydrogen peroxide solution that would take out the bloodstains before they set. Since I had blood on me, the television cameras, hungry for interesting pictures, swung in my direction. They were still focused on me cleaning up at the back of the van when two shots rang out. I cursed at myself for not wearing my bulletproof vest on a hot day and hit the deck, as did nearly everyone else in sight, except of course for the two corn-fed, young female PAs-in-training. Being from the rural Midwest, they did not recognize the sound of a gun firing in an urban setting, and I yanked them down beside me.

Then I heard a car door slam shut and a car peel away. I continued to listen, but heard no more shots. Although it seemed almost inconceivable, another murder had just taken place, this time in front of three hundred witnesses, as well as thirty or forty police officials and at least three television news crews. After I ascertained that no more shots were coming, I headed across the street, in the direction from which the sounds had come.

The shooter was already gone, having jumped into a waiting car to escape, but here was the new victim, sagging on the sidewalk, in the process of expiring. I rushed toward him, thinking perhaps that I might attempt resuscitative efforts, but one look at the very large holes in the center of his chest told me that this young man was not going to need my rusty clinical skills. He expired before I actually reached his side.

I was kneeling at the body, perhaps ten seconds later, when a plainclothes cop came over, holding out his old-fashioned six-shooter, pointed toward the sky in a ready position in case the bad guy came back. I recognized the plainclothes cop from previous cases: a deputy police chief in charge of Manhattan North's detective division. He looked down at me, and at the body, and quipped, "Great response time from the ME's office."

Later I learned that the third victim was believed to be the rival gang member who had shot the two in the stairwell and had foolishly gone back to the scene of the crime to watch the hullabaloo. Apparently, as he was gloating, a member of the first victim's gang had taken revenge for their deaths.

This was not the only time I heard shots fired while out on a case or the only time that those shots resulted in my next scene investigation. The homicide rate in the city was skyrocketing, and we at the OCME were being pushed to our limits in dealing with it. For five years in the early to middle 1990s, I put in an average of eighty hours a week as an MLI-II: The crack epidemic was making the city's homicide rate soar to more than two thousand a year, but at the same time the city was under a hiring freeze, which prevented OCME from hiring more MLIs to handle our large caseload.

The three victims in the "stairwell-and-sidewalk" case were casualties of that crack epidemic.

Crack cocaine is a terrifyingly addictive drug that is, unfortunately, easy and cheap to make. It produces walking zombies, burned-out people. Studies have shown that a person can become addicted after taking a *single* dose. During those years of the mid-1990s, we would often be summoned to a crack house, an abandoned building, warehouse, or apartment that had become the location where crack addicts obtained and used their poison—and where, on a regular basis, they perished. In earlier eras, there had been opium dens, but compared to crack houses those opium dens had been orderly, controlled, still-human places. Everything in a crack house that could be sold for money had been sold, so inside there was usually no electricity, no heat, no light, no furniture except for a moldy mattress or two, and, likely as not, no intact windows. You entered a crack house and smelled immediately the mingled scents of urine, feces, vomit, sweat, and despair. There we would find emaciated bodies of addicts dead from overdoses, violence, malnutrition, or diseases that could have been treated but instead had been neglected.

Once, we found an addict's body in an advanced stage of decomposition in a public housing stairwell; the housing authority police swore that it had not been there the previous day, when they had done their "vertical patrol," so we had to assume it had come from some interior, crack-house apartment, and that its stench had finally become too much for the other denizens. This was not difficult to believe, as often the bodies found inside the crack houses had obviously been there for quite some time before anyone was motivated enough to alert authorities to their presence.

The combination of crack/heroin-addled junkies and cigarette lighters makes for a combustible mixture, and every now and then a drug den would go up in flames. Most of the fires were accidental, but sometimes not. On one occasion, I was called to the scene of a fire in a supposedly empty, four-story, walk-up building near Harlem Hospital. The fire department, in the process of putting out the blaze, had discovered a victim, burned beyond recognition, in a second-floor room. Already uptown for another case, I was able to respond within minutes of receiving the call, and arrived to join a meeting, outside the building, of local precinct detectives, fire marshals, and the fire chief in charge. Fire marshals are firefighters who, after serving for a number of years with a regular fire company, have taken additional specialized training in fire investigation. They have police powers and carry guns, and in New York City their jurisdiction extends over all arson-related crimes, including homicides.

Louie Garcia, a field supervisor in the fire marshals unit, gave me the rundown. "One body, charred, second floor; building was condemned but it looks like addicts got in and were using the place for a while." Along with the detectives, Louie and his fire marshal partner, and the fire chief, I trooped upstairs. The risers on the stairs had burned through, so we walked up by stepping on a turgid fire hose that had been run up the stairs. Smoke was still drifting off the walls, and when we reached the second floor, one of the detectives, in a show of bravado, lit a cigarette off a red-hot metal wall stud. As we neared the body, it was clear that the fire had begun on or around it. The flame and burn patterns pointed out to me by Louie indicated that an accelerant, probably gasoline, had been poured over the body and that the fire had spread from there. The floor under the victim appeared pretty burned through, so I asked the fire chief, "Will that floor hold me?" He replied by stamping his foot hard on the floor and grinning.

I approached the body, and just as I leaned over it to begin my examination the entire ceiling above me gave way and came crashing down, knocking me to the floor and directly onto the burned corpse. I was covered in about a foot of plaster and burned wood, but luckily no real heavy chunks hit me.

My colleagues dug me out, and as I straightened up, the fire chief held his hands out as if to deny responsibility and said, "Hey, you asked me about the floor!"

I was okay, so we all had a good laugh and I returned to the business at hand, which was to confirm that this was indeed a homicide. From my on-scene investigation, I was able to determine that the victim had been shot at least three times in the chest.

An autopsy the next day revealed that he had died before the fire was started. Despite the ceiling mishap, I bore no grudge against the fire department, and Louie Garcia and I became fast friends. Over the years, I was pleased to watch Louie's steady climb to the top job of chief fire marshal for New York City.

During the crack epidemic, a rather chilling phrase came into common use among the members of New York's criminal justice fraternity—"misdemeanor homicide." A misdemeanor, of course, is a crime that is not serious enough to be a felony; the phrase misdemeanor homicide denotes a murder that the cops would not treat seriously, such as one in which two crackheads gunned down each other. In those years, the city was averaging six homicides a day, of which maybe three were crack related. It was a soul-numbing parade of violence, and after a few years on the job, I understood why the overworked police did not want to treat all homicides with equal seriousness. I first heard the term in East New York, Brooklyn, on Mother Gaston Boulevard—this plague of homicides often took me beyond Manhattan. A plainclothes police lieutenant, a detective, used the phrase in casual conversation with other cops at a scene at which a drug dealer had been mowed down in a hail of gunfire from an Uzi submachine gun. The phrase made its way into popular culture in 1993, when a fictional detective in the television show *Homicide: Life on the Street* said the line, "Baltimore, home of the misdemeanor homicide." I am not sure in which city the phrase was actually coined, but in New York, it became so widely used that it provoked an edict from City Hall: no one who worked for the city, as a cop or in any other capacity, was to use the phrase, ever. It was considered demeaning and racist since the overwhelming majority of the victims of the crack epidemic were black or Latino.

Abolishing the use of that particularly offensive term did not mean that every homicide was treated the same. During the heyday of the crack epidemic, there were just too many homicides for the police to give them each a full court press. Friends of mine in the NYPD privately confirmed what I was seeing at death scenes—cases were unofficially triaged, and detective bosses decided which to investigate based on the case's apparent solvability and on the identity of the victim. Simply put, the murder investigation of an Upper East Side investment banker would of course be the beneficiary of more resources and attention than the murder of a street hood with twelve prior narcotics arrests.

The city denied then that any such triage existed and blustered on about how dedicated civil servants devoted equal attention to every crime, big or small, and every victim, rich or poor, minority or majority. Such protestations made for good sound bites but simply did not reflect reality. However, I must note that as the homicide rate in New York City dropped, through the remainder of the decade and on into the twenty-first century, to record lows, there was an increasingly more equitable distribution of attention to homicides.

While the NYPD may have been able to unofficially shrug off any particular death, in the 1990s, OCME could not then, and cannot ever do so. Perhaps the difference is a function of our respective mandates. Remember, cops focus primarily on the *perpetrator* and on the questions: *Who did it?* and *Why?* We at OCME focus on the *victim: Who is dead?* and *What happened?* Each death therefore must be treated by us with the same care, attention to detail, and dignity as any other. This difference of focus is a further reiteration of the status of OCME as not being a part of law *enforcement,* though one of OCME's functions is indeed to support the criminal justice system. Its other duties are to support the public health system and the civil legal structure—the latter, for instance, coming into play when an ME testifies in a civil case, or, more frequently, in the issuing of the death certificate that is necessary to the proper processing of the decedent's estate.

The "misdemeanor homicide" brouhaha also brings to mind that our designation of the manner of death as a homicide sometimes causes problems for the police. We must call any death *purposefully* brought about by the hands of another person a homicide, even if there is no attendant criminality. Sometimes this legal requirement drives cops crazy. Take, for an exaggerated example, an instance in which a bank robber shoots his way out of a bank, only to encounter outside a phalanx of police and circling media, all alerted by the bank's silent alarm. Despite appropriate warnings given by the police to drop his weapon, the robber decides to try to shoot his way through the cordon and is met by a hail of police bullets that ends his life. All of the action is recorded by the impartial media, with the result that there was never a more open-and-shut case of a "justifiable shooting." Even so, OCME must still label this death a homicide. And because we do, a grand jury will have to be empanelled to consider whether the homicide is, as the police will argue, a justifiable one. That it is justifiable will probably take the grand jury only a few moments to determine. But OCME has to call it a homicide and issue a death certificate that lists homicide as the manner of death. There is simply no other choice for us.

Should New York State ever enforce its death penalty, and if the resulting execution takes place in New York City, OCME will issue the death certificate, and I guarantee that the manner of death will be listed as homicide. This is the major reason that I am firmly against the death penalty. Despite all of the deadly violence that I have witnessed or perhaps because of it, I am against murder of any kind. This is not to say that I'm soft on criminals; on the contrary, I am a firm believer in life without parole truly meaning life without parole. That is fitting retributive justice for committing the sorts of homicides I saw way too often in my years as a medicolegal investigator.

In the early 1990s, the crack epidemic was its own death penalty for far too many victims, some of them much too young to have merited execution by the poison and the violence it spawned. In order to keep up with the death toll, I sometimes worked three shifts in a row, not because I wanted to but because every other MLI was also busy with the caseload. Now and then, on the midnight-to-eight shift, we could cat-nap until the phone rang. Still further on into the crack epidemic, the office decided that on our third shift in a row, if it was an overnight, a slow time for death reports, we could stay at home and only respond when calls came in. Later, that stay-at-home policy was disallowed by the city, in response to a perceived scandal in which some MLIs were shown to be taking home more money in a year because of overtime pay than the mayor and other top officials earned. The tabloids had a field day when my fellow MLI Joe Savino earned so much in overtime that he made more than the president of the United States. The *New York Post* published a list of the city's top overtime earners, with Joey as number one. I was no slouch that year, coming in at number four or five, but I received little media attention—that was reserved for Joey. Much of the attention was negative. The city's Department of Investigation began to look into the overtime "scandal." They found no illegalities because there were none to find. Joey Savino put in so many hours talking to doctors about the deaths that occurred in their hospitals that in one Bronx hospital, when someone died in the ER, they would say that the patient had "done a Savino."

At that point, OCME was simply understaffed and overworked; there were twelve investigators doing the job that today is done by forty. And in those days, we MLIs handled more then four times the current annual load of murders. Sometimes, in the mid-1990s, it seemed to me that I was always working; and when I was tired, say toward the end of a double shift, I'd think to myself, "Well, at least my patients are already dead." At such moments, out at a scene and knowing that my judgment was not at its best, I'd often just have the body brought into the OCME house, so we could look at it in the morning, when we were all fresh.

105

It was during these hectic years that the hours and demand of my job began to have consequences beyond the office. As I tried to stay grounded throughout the trials of my work, I found that my relationship with my wife, and my religion, were growing strained. My faith would ebb and flow in reaction to my shifting moods and constantly evolving beliefs about Orthodox Judaism. During that same period, partially due to my dissatisfaction with Orthodoxy, and partially due to the huge amounts of overtime that I was putting in, my first marriage crumbled and my wife and I divorced. She remained within the Orthodox community, while I continued the process of leaving it. The divorce and my diminishing adherence to Orthodox doctrine put a tremendous strain on my relationship with my birth family.

I was learning painfully the extent to which my job would take its toll. Such was the nature of my life with other people's deaths.

SEVEN

WORKING A TON of hours as an MLI and handling many cases, I got to know a lot of cops. I came to recognize most of the detectives working in Manhattan and a fair number of the uniformed officers too, but even more of them seemed to know who I was or at least where I worked. That was logical because during the homicide heyday of the early 1990s, we MLIs were working many hours and cases and there were fewer of us than there were police detectives. Everywhere I went, I'd bump into some police officer, either a uniform or a detective, who would say, "Hi, doc."

Once, on my way to visit a sick friend, I was walking along a street on Manhattan's Upper West Side. I was out of my customary work uniform—a dark suit, braces, white shirt, tie, and polished black shoes. Like NYPD detectives, most MLIs dress in business attire when out in the field, but since I was not on the schedule that day, I was wearing my off-duty uniform: jeans, sweatshirt, and sneakers.

As I walked along, I noticed out of the corner of my eye that an NYPD patrol car was pacing me. I walked a little faster, and it matched my speed. I slowed and so did the car. Getting a little paranoid, I crossed the street and started walking the opposite way. They flipped on their overhead lights and made an illegal turn across a double yellow, caught up with me, turned off their lights and kept pacing me. Feeling a little like a wanted man, I turned toward the police car, ready to surrender, and got my first really good look inside of it: two of New

York City's Finest, laughing their heads off. As I drew nearer, I recognized the pair of jokers from dozens of death scenes that we had worked together.

"Okay, you two, what gives?" I demanded.

"Well, doc," one of them said through his laughter, "we just wanted to see what an ME did on his day off, so we followed you—but it was a good six blocks before you noticed us!" I pretended that this was funny and joked with them for a few moments before going on my way.

Sure, it was funny. But this was also a significant moment because it demonstrated to me that the cops had finally come to accept the MLIs—not necessarily as their own, but as people they could have fun with. For the first time I could see a level of acceptance that meant they'd made room for me on their side of the Thin Blue Line. The MLI corps had only been around for a few years and cops have always lived by tradition. While their initial skepticism about this new breed of ME investigator often led them to doubt our abilities, as time went on, they (and the DAs) became impressed with our technically expert performances at scenes. It was also our sharing of their social interactions—going to the same retirement parties and attending the same lectures and conventions—that eventually paved the way for us to become accepted partners in New York's criminal justice community.

The more comfortable the NYPD became with our crime scene roles, the more we were able to take on roles that were not ordinarily prescribed for MLIs. These special relationships that we seasoned MLIs developed with the members of the police force sometimes took us a bit far afield of our usual endeavors as death investigators. In just this way, I came to be asked to do something highly unusual for an MLI: go undercover. My friends on the force thought the particular situation called for someone with my . . . talents.

The detective squad at the First Precinct had received word that a set of "babies in bottles," preserved fetuses, were going to be auctioned off at a "nature" or "curio" store in Lower Manhattan. The detectives wanted me to get a look at the preserved remains and to determine if they were really human. If so, the next step would be to figure out whether this proposed auction was legal. To the cops, it seemed that selling the preserved bodies of human babies should be illegal; as one detective opined, "it just feels wrong." I assured them that if the remains were human, it was very likely that selling them was illegal. But before we brought this to the DA's office, we agreed that I should go in undercover, posing as a potential buyer to assess what was really in those bottles.

The back story was this: For many years, an abortionist in Florida had collected fetuses as part of his work and had chosen to preserve some of them with formaldehyde, storing them in large glass jars. He had evidently intended to create a panoramic display that showed every stage of the development of a human being *in utero,* from microscopic to full term, and when completed, to donate the collection to a medical school. At the time of his death, he had accumulated a nearly complete set of sixty or so fetuses, stored in a number of large jars. However, someone executing the doctor's estate had chosen not to donate the fetuses but to sell them—to a traveling freak show.

Eventually, that traveling freak show came to Brooklyn's Coney Island, and there alongside the bearded lady, the midget, and the inevitable fat man, the jarred fetuses were put on display. An offended patron (who obviously drew the line of good taste at preserved babies) phoned in a disgusted complaint to his local police precinct. The OCME was eventually called, but by the time my Brooklyn colleagues arrived at where the show was supposed to be located, it had packed up and moved on.

Shortly thereafter, the police learned that the preserved fetuses had turned up again and now were in Manhattan and were about to be auctioned off by the curio shop on Spring Street. This was when my police friends persuaded me to go into the shop, undercover, as a potential buyer of the fetuses.

I had actually been to the store before. It was a legitimate place of business, chock-full of preserved insects, animal-hide rugs, fossils, meteorite fragments, bones, and other assorted knickknacks. It was one of the few places in the city where you could purchase a full-size replica of a human skull or even a fully articulated human skeleton. It billed itself as an "oasis for children," and, indeed, kids loved to browse around the aisles and cluster around the shark teeth and preserved alligator heads.

As undercover debuts go, this one was—for me, at least—disappointingly tame. I did not wear a wire (hidden recording device), and no backup waited in unmarked cars outside in case the operation went bad. I entered the store, found the owner, and inquired if it was true that he had some babies in jars for sale. He did not attempt to conceal this, nor did he ask me any questions that might have betrayed some nervousness at selling the jars and their contents. He took me downstairs to the storage area, where he showed me a few jars holding the well-preserved remains of what were clearly human fetuses, some of whom were obviously full-term babies. Hiding my shock, I talked to the owner for a few moments and gained the impression that he felt that there was nothing wrong in selling these human remains. He indicated to me that he considered the babies to be anatomical specimens, much like the preserved baby sharks that were for sale upstairs. I declined to buy a baby-in-a-jar that day, and to allay suspicion, I browsed aimlessly around the store for a few more moments before leaving.

Using my report, the cops raided the place, confiscated the specimens and brought them to the ME's office where Mark Flomenbaum, the first deputy Chief Medical Examiner, looked them over. Mark agreed with my field assessment that at least five of the fetuses were near- or full-term babies. The shop owner was eventually arrested and charged with a series of crimes ranging from mishandling hazardous materials (the formalin) to illegal possession of and attempted sale of human remains.

I don't know the outcome of the case against the owner, but I do know that the preserved babies were eventually donated to a medical school. I was happy to have played a small but critical part in this crime-busting endeavor.

By this time, I had been working at the ME's office for a number of years, and since much of the crushing workload of the early years had subsided, I started to have some time to myself after my usual workweek came to a close. I had grown concerned that my clinical skills were deteriorating to the point that I would never be able to return to clinical practice, so I began looking for a part-time clinical position where I could work a few shifts a month and hone my clinical abilities. Glancing through the newspaper, I came across an advertisement for a job that seemed perfect. An inner-city clinic, located in the Bronx and quite similar to the one where I began my career, was seeking PAs for shift work. I called up the clinic, faxed in my credentials, and was asked to come to meet the owner, a man I'll call Michael Smith.

From our first meeting, he was incredibly forthcoming about what he was doing. He had hooked up with a retired psychiatrist in the Bronx and was planning to use that psychiatrist's license number to write prescriptions and to submit the bills to Medicaid and Medicare. Smith, whom I came to realize had no medical degree and no experience in clinical medicine, even though he walked around in a long white coat that read "Michael Smith, MD, Trauma Surgeon," told me that together we could make enormous amounts of money, seeing patients at the clinic on Webster Avenue and maybe even opening additional clinics. After the interview, he took me to City Island and onto his yacht, a fifty-footer, the largest boat, other than a cruise ship, on which I had ever set foot. He wined and dined me and treated me as though I was the answer to his prayers.

I went home and turned the events over in my mind, eventually deciding to call a friend who was an assistant DA. He put me in touch with the Medicaid/Medicare fraud unit at the New York State Attorney General's office, and I arranged a meeting there, walked in, and started telling my story. As soon as I mentioned the name Michael Smith, I could see they were interested and that they already knew this guy.

At the suggestion of the AG's investigators, I returned to the clinic and "worked" a couple of shifts that were agony for me. Many of the patients I saw were quite ill, and as word got out that someone in the clinic was actually listening to patients and, presumably, treating them (actually I was deliberately *not* treating them to prevent any potentially illegal action on my part), the waiting room became crowded, and lines started to form outside the clinic. These patients broke my heart. They were the poorest of the poor. They would plaintively ask, with hope in their voices, "Are you going to be my doctor now?" Many were quite ill, needing medications. One told me he hadn't been able to afford blood pressure medication for two years, so he hadn't taken any in that time and his pressure was through the roof. Smith stalked around the place in his white coat, stethoscope, and phony ID badge that announced he was a "trauma surgeon," but saw no patients himself. He confided once again, during that day, his plan to open other clinics all over the Bronx and his offer that if I stuck with him, we were going to be rich.

My job, for the AG's office, was to get Smith to act as though he was a physician supervising my work. Since I absolutely could not treat patients or write prescriptions for them, all I did was talk with them and take their histories. I did not even give them advice. I couldn't, or else I'd be part of the scheme, too. My frustration was palpable, and being unable to help people suffering from such treatable illnesses was utter torture.

After my two shifts, I was debriefed by the AG's office, who then prepared to go in, arrest Smith for, among other things, practicing medicine without a license, and close the operation.

I was never sure about what happened next, because the AG's office did not keep me in the loop, but I do know that Smith got away. Somehow, he either got word of the impending raid, or figured out that I had been a plant, and decided to decamp. He went aboard his yacht, slipped the moorings, sailed off, and has not been heard from again. As far as I know, he was never prosecuted, but that particular Medicaid mill was closed; and this intrepid undercover went back to work in the ME's office, somewhat the worse for wear.

While these undercover operations constituted the extent of my time working on the enforcement side of the law, my career continued to produce encounters with the DA's office. When I received my promotion to MLI-II, it meant more than just being able to work without supervision; it also meant that I had finally reached the level where it was acceptable for me to testify in criminal court cases. While it would seem to be a fairly routine responsibility for an investigator, in truth, this was a serious matter with consequences that would reflect on not just my reputation and that of the OCME but also on the defendant's freedom and the ultimate justice for the victim.

Before testifying in court for the first time, I was filled with nervous anticipation. Waiting outside the courtroom to be called as a witness, I felt my hands go cold and my mouth dry up. I expected to enter a perfectly groomed courtroom, with dark wood-paneled walls and vaulted ceilings, where no less than Clarence Darrow would speak for the defense, and *Law & Order*'s Jack McCoy would represent the prosecution; for the judge, I pictured in my mind's eye a stern yet lovable Fred Gwynne, reprising his judicial role in the movie *My Cousin Vinny*.

After arriving at that first courtroom, my expectations were mightily disappointed. To my inexperienced eye, the hall of justice seemed shabby, and the judge, lawyers, and other staffers appeared bored and perfunctory in the exercise of arcane rituals that I mostly couldn't follow. Over the years, though, by taking part in and observing many trials, I learned that while most of New York's real-life courtrooms are nowhere near as well appointed as the courts seen in *Law & Order*, and while the personnel staffing them may not be as exciting to watch, they get the job done. I understood why the Manhattan DA's office ranks among the best in the United States and learned that what I had mistaken for perfunctory effort was actually a display of competent professionalism, as the assistant DAs went through the innumerable steps necessary to bring an alleged perpetrator to justice.

In that first trial, I was called as a Fact Witness, testifying to the provenance of blood I had drawn for DNA testing. In New York County courts (and, I am sure, in most other jurisdictions), in order to have an object or record admitted into evidence, its pedigree or provenance—from whence it came—must be demonstrated. This means that someone has to say, under oath, or be otherwise able to prove, where the evidence came from, and where it has been, each step of the way, from the moment it was found until this very moment when the evidence is being offered to the court. Often there is a chain-of-custody record, and it suffices. But many times, establishing the pedigree of a particular piece of evidence requires witness testimony, and that was to be my job in this first trial.

The night before I was to testify, I was sleepless, imagining the fierce barrage of questions I would receive from the pitiless defense attorney. In truth, my debut was straightforward and matter-of-fact. It went like this: "Yes, I drew that blood, I gave the blood to that detective, and yes, that's my signature on the envelope seal." The evidence was admitted into the record, and I was dismissed without as much as a raised eyebrow from the defense attorney. I left the courtroom with a new perspective on my relative importance in the grand design of the criminal justice system.

Of course, getting physical evidence admitted into a trial isn't the only thing done by Fact Witnesses. Actually, most of the testimony in ordinary trials is delivered by Fact Witnesses who say such factual things as "I saw Johnny shoot Jimmy." Fact Witnesses testify to what they saw, or heard, or know to be true because they have first-hand knowledge of it. What Fact Witnesses do not do, cannot do, is render an *opinion*. That privilege is reserved for the Expert Witness.

Later on, as a natural result of my MLI-II work on a case, I was called by the DA's office to testify for the first time as an Expert Witness. The prosecutor needed my testimony about the victim's time of death so that he could then elicit testimony that would place the defendant at the scene at around that same time. But for me to testify as an expert, since I had never done so before, I would first have to be qualified. This would occur, during the trial, in front of a jury; the process is called *voir dire*. In it, the prosecutor would present me and explain to the court why I should be permitted to testify as an expert. The defense attorney would also have an opportunity to try to discredit me, and thus prevent me from testifying or leave a doubt in the minds of the jurors as to what I would say when testifying.

To my surprise, I was not nearly as nervous as I had been prior to my testifying the first time as a Fact Witness. Perhaps that was because, by this point, I had given testimony in a number of trials, or perhaps it was due to my feeling of confidence that I was, by now, indeed, quite an expert in my job. The prosecutor elicited my experience through his questioning: my training in medicine as a PA, my training at the ME's office as an MLI-I, and my independent work as an MLI-II who had already, I testified, investigated hundreds if not a thousand death scenes.

Then, the defense attorney, as I had expected him to, challenged my credentials, and I raised the ante, saying that I had already investigated more homicides in my relatively brief career as an MLI than most homicide detectives do in their entire careers.

He was unable to dispute that, but in his parting shot at me, the defense attorney uttered something like, "Yeah, yeah . . . but you're not a doctor."

I know an opening when I see one. Did this attorney think he was the first person to needle this nice Jewish boy from Brooklyn about not being a doctor? "No, I'm not a doctor, but you're not a doctor either," I responded.

The jury guffawed, and I think even the judge chuckled, but he cautioned me to confine myself to responding to the questions, not to commenting.

"Respectfully, judge, I am being responsive. My point is that this attorney does not need to be a doctor to do what he does, and I don't need to be a doctor to do what I do. In fact, I am fully qualified to do what I do. The city's administrative code says that MLIs are to be PAs, and I have all the proper training and credentials to perform as an MLI-II. The job is specifically made for a PA and not for a doctor."

At this point, the judge qualified me as an expert with no further questioning. He also instructed the jury that I was an expert, that they were to consider my testimony as they would that of any other expert, and that they were not to hold it against me that this was the first time I'd be testifying as an Expert Witness.

Thereafter, I testified as an Expert Witness in a number of cases. In a few, I provided crucial testimony that helped lead to a conviction—for instance, in the case that Perry Mason would no doubt refer to as the "box of diapers" homicide.

The incident took place at a bodega (a neighborhood convenience store), and began just after midnight in the Washington Heights section of Manhattan, when a new father was sent out of his apartment by his wife to buy diapers for their infant. He went to the bodega and found one lone box of Pampers on a shelf. He grabbed it. Another customer in the store claimed that it was his box to buy, that he had just put it down for a second while fetching a soft drink. The two fathers quarreled. The soda-grabber left the store, but came back a few moments later, aimed a gun at the new father, who was by then at the register with the diapers, and killed him with a single shot to the head.

When I arrived, I found the decedent lying near the counter, his body angled away from the door, and an undisturbed pool of blood surrounding his head on the floor. The box of Pampers was still on the counter, waiting for checkout. The employee behind the counter told the cops the story of the altercation, and what I found while examining the scene corroborated his account and more.

The shooter was soon arrested and charged with murder.

I was asked by the DA's office to testify at his trial. Although it had seemed to me earlier like an open-and-shut case, what with the physical evidence and the testimony of the store employee, it was not because the defense was arguing that the shooter had killed the new father in self-defense. The shooter's attorney contended that either the police or EMS had moved the body to the position in which it had been found— that the decedent had actually been shot closer to the door, where the alleged struggle had taken place, and had later been moved to the site next to the counter and cash register.

Given what I've conveyed earlier in this book about EMS's willingness to disturb a homicide scene in a vain attempt to resuscitate a dead body, there could have been good reason to accept the defense's contentions. However, the evidence did not support the defense's contention. Having done my work at the death scene carefully, I was able to show in the courtroom, with the aid of photographic blow-ups and diagrams, what had actually happened in the bodega. If you stood the father up, I told the jury, you would find him at the counter, with his body turned in the direction of the door, where the shooter had entered. He had fallen directly backward under the impact of the bullet.

In addition, there were no powder burns on the decedent's clothing—which meant that he and the shooter had been at least thirty-six inches apart—providing evidence that they had *not* struggled and that the shooter had been far enough away so that he did not have to defend himself against the new father's purported attack.

I also demonstrated other evidence from the scene that further belied the shooter's claim of self-defense. There were no bloodstains close to the door, where they would have had to be if there had been a struggle. The only blood (aside from modest spatter on the aisle behind the decedent) was pooled under the victim's head, which similarly argued against the body having been moved by the cops or EMTs. Finally I showed the jury that the pool of blood beneath and around the victim's head had perfect margins and told them that once such a pool is formed, it cannot be disturbed and then put back together again without breaking the meniscus (the almost invisible but palpable outer shell of a liquid). "You can't collect blood and push it back into shape," I said to the jury. "It smears." I asked them to recall seeing drops of their own blood fall from finger-pricks or other injuries; those drops remain intact until disturbed, but once violated, they couldn't be moved without smearing.

With those words, the jury understood that the new father could not have died while attacking the shooter, rejected the defendant's claim of self-defense, and convicted him of murder.

Frequently, the beginner MLI-IIs are handed the cases that appear to be routine and don't require a veteran's eye for detail. While this was initially the drill for me, as I became a more experienced and seasoned MLI-II, more of the curious and unusual death scenes came my way.

On one such occasion, I was called to a pizzeria that was located on a busy crosstown street in mid-Manhattan. The owners had decided to make a backyard palazzo for outdoor dining, and the contractor whom they hired to dig up the spot had soon turned up bones—lots of bones. Gigantic bones, some twenty to thirty inches long and nine to ten inches in diameter. Bones so big that the contractor and the restaurateurs thought they might belong to dinosaurs.

Though these remains were clearly not human, the drill in New York City is, if you find bones, you call the ME's office. Summoned to the scene by police, I was immediately able to verify the bones were not human. And our anthropologist was later able to confirm that they belonged to a large species of hog.

One of the basic facts about Manhattan is that each building site has been used for four or five different purposes in the city's nearly four centuries of existence. Examining the historical records of the building, we shortly learned that at the turn of the twentieth century, the restaurant's site had been the location of a butcher shop. Evidently the butcher had carved up the hogs on the site and buried the meatless bones in the backyard. I was told that the cache of bones went down twenty feet.

The owners of the pizzeria, I think, must have been disappointed that the bones were not those of dinosaurs, whose presence might have added a certain cachet to the palazzo.

In truth, finding bones in New York City is not that unique. Whether they're left out on the street or buried in the ground, they seem to turn up regularly. Perhaps the most amusing bone case I was ever called out on involved a collection of bones found on the street in a black plastic bag. Recently, a dead baby had been discovered in such a bag on a New York street, and the tabloids and the local television news were full of the tragedy. And, as often happens when something of that nature is publicized, in the weeks after the event, people's eyes were sharpened for such an occurrence, and we got many calls on similar-looking problems.

It was another one of those blistering hot days in the city. A small crowd had gathered, kept from an area near the side of a building by yellow tape. I found a rookie cop, as usual, sitting alongside the bag of bones, sweating, nervous, and glad to see me. His look told me that he thought this could be a homicide—which would mean lots of paperwork and other botheration.

I opened the bag, stuck in my gloved hand, and pulled out a bone. It was large and could have been a section of thighbone, but I wasn't certain. However, the bone was covered with a certain dark brown patina, as though it had been painted with shellac, and it had a peculiar odor. I pulled out a few more bones of similar size, and they all had the same odor and patina. The rookie cop, curious, had edged quite close to me.

I turned to him and said, "If this is a homicide, then we're looking for Emeril Lagasse."

He didn't get the joke, so I explained. The Food Network show host and star chef uses a lot of hickory smoking in his barbecue and other preparations in his cooking. The bones in this instance, too, had been smoked with hickory—not for human taste buds, however, but for the delectation of dogs. I had seen many similar cases: each year, we actually receive a number of similar calls in which large bones, usually bovine, are dumped on the street, usually after a dog has chewed them.

I always kept an open mind, though, because the bones did not always turn out to be cattle. One day we received a call about a finding of bones that sent me out to Governor's Island. This island, off the south end of Manhattan, was then owned by the federal government and used by the Coast Guard. To reach it, you had to take a ferry from Lower Manhattan, which I did—a nice trip on a nice day. The island is an historic site. It has several complexes of buildings on it, including an old fort and even a small nine-hole golf course. There were also a number of parking lots, and the Coast Guard had been digging a trench for an electrical conduit through one such paved-over parking lot when they turned up some human-looking bones and called the police. (Even though a Coast Guard facility is federal property, the local police and OCME have jurisdiction over dead bodies.) Naturally the police called us, and when I debarked the ferry, I was met by Frank Libby, a Coast Guard chief warrant officer, who escorted me over to the site and filled me in on how the bones had come to be found.

The hole in the parking lot was quite long and about four feet deep, and I spent several hours hanging upside down, looking into it, brushing soil away from the bones and gingerly exposing them. They were, indeed, human bones and from more than one body. Upon closer inspection, it became obvious to me that these bones were not modern. There were no coffins; either there had never been any or they had rotted away long ago. There was no dental work on the teeth in the skulls, which placed the period of the deaths before modern dentistry. Augmenting that notion was a long-barreled, small-chambered pipe that I found near the bones, which looked to be Dutch—after all, New York had once been Nieuw Amsterdam, and Governor's Island had been one of the first Dutch outposts here. With these clues in hand, I dubbed the remains archaeological and suggested that the Coast Guard have a museum look into them.

The Museum of Natural History was called, and their staff eventually took quite a few skeletons from the trench. The bones were determined to have most likely come from a Dutch hospital on the site in the 1600s, possibly the victims of tuberculosis or another wasting disease.

EIGHT

AFTER A FEW years as an MLI-II, I became a senior or supervising MLI. This new designation was an in-house title only, since the city had not yet gotten around to creating the actual title of MLI-III. Official or not, in this capacity I was responsible for supervising the work of the MLI-Is, scheduling all of the Manhattan MLIs, training newly hired MLIs and MEs, and acting as a clinical "preceptor" to the droves of residents, medical students, and PA students who rotated through our office. Last but not least, I was also getting to handle some interesting and unusual cases.

One of these didn't initially present as all that unusual to the detectives who first investigated it. The death scene was in a high-rise apartment building that had been undergoing renovation. A handyman had been installing dishwashers in a line of apartments up and down the building, and as he was installing the ninth dishwasher that day, he died, right under the sink. A few hours later, the construction foreman overseeing the renovations found him and called 911. EMS pronounced him dead at the scene. And even though they did not attempt CPR (because he was already exhibiting rigor mortis), they did—as usual—disturb the scene by pulling him out from under the sink. The NYPD detectives, learning from the EMT that the body had no visible trauma, concluded that the death was from a heart attack, and left the scene. When I looked around, I felt there was just something wrong with this judgment. Over the years, I'd developed what old-hand MLIs call "scene instinct," which in this instance was reminding me that natural heart attack death scenes *feel* different from those of workplace accidents. And this one felt like the latter.

There were several clues. The decedent had been a relatively young man, in his forties, and he was slender and appeared to be in good physical condition—not a likely heart attack victim. Moreover, he had died *under* the sink; even people who have suffered massive heart attacks usually have enough strength and time left to stagger out of such confined spaces before they succumb.

Going through my usual routine, I went over the scene, examined the body, and found nothing. Nevertheless my inner alarm bells would not stop ringing. Something was wrong here, and I needed to find out what that was. To put an end to my lingering doubt, I did something that I would not have been able to do when I was a more junior MLI-II: I used my senior status to ask my colleague Nick Fusco to come out to the scene. Nick was not an MLI or an ME but an architect who served as OCME's facilities manager. By my work, I had, I believe, earned enough respect from him that he agreed to meet me at the death scene.

Soon after he arrived at the scene, he ratified my guess that this was no natural death. He took apart the dishwasher, and in doing so, discovered that when the handyman was wiring the dishwasher into the wall, he had "juiced the ground." In other words, the handyman had electrically grounded the machine the wrong way, ensuring that if he touched both the exterior metal case of the dishwasher, and something else that was metal or conductive, he would complete an electrical circuit through his own body and electrocute himself.

Nick suggested that I examine the body for signs of electrocution. There were no outward signs on the body, except for a slightly suspicious mark high on the shoulder where it met the neck. After Nick made the area safe, I crawled under the sink and arranged myself into the position in which the foreman said he found the body. In that cramped position under the sink, I found that my neck was pressed against the waste pipe of the sink. With my right hand, I reached out and could easily touch the outside of the dishwasher. These must have been the two points through which the handyman's body had created a circuit: hand on the dishwasher, neck on the damp waste pipe under the sink . . . and ZAP! But this was still a guess on my part. To obtain more information, the body had to be taken back to the OCME and its tissues put under a microscope.

When we used the microscope to examine what lay underneath the bruised skin of the neck area, the cells there displayed *nuclear streaming*—the nuclei were not in their usual circular central position in the cells but rather appeared in an elongated position and were lined up facing in a single direction rather than in the usual random pattern. This is why the condition is known as streaming. It is a hallmark of electrocution.

Based on these findings, we were able to rule that the handyman had died from accidental electrocution, but our job wasn't finished. We went back to the apartment building and, sure enough, found that all of the other recently installed dishwashers had been wired in the same dangerously wrong way, and if they were left that way, they could have eventually electrocuted the tenants. We saw to it that all of the building's dishwashers were properly rewired by a licensed electrician. The handyman who had been installing the dishwashers had not been a licensed electrician, and his ignorance of proper procedure had cost him his life.

We took some satisfaction from our sleuthing and prevention work in the dishwasher case, and my friend Nick was proud to add to his business card the phrase "Forensic Architect."

The case was concluded, but two aspects of it continued to bother me. Why hadn't the cops investigated the possibility that the handyman's death had been something other than a natural death? More important, why had they accepted the EMS's assertion that there was no trauma and used that as license to leave the scene? I could only conclude that the cops had been primarily interested in finding out whodunit and establishing whether there had been foul play. Once the detectives in this case had concluded there was no foul play, and thus no perp to chase and collar, they had lost interest.

I was much more bothered by the lack of assigned *responsibility* for the handyman's death. OCME issued a death certificate ruling the death accidental, and certainly it could be argued that the handyman's death was his own fault and no one else was to blame. But I thought this death had occurred in circumstances that warranted broader investigation. To my knowledge, no police or other authorities investigated whether the owner of the building had tried to keep expenses down by hiring an unlicensed handyman to install the dishwashers rather than using a licensed (and more expensive) electrician. Part of the problem was that no *existing* investigative body had the proper mandate to look into this death. Only on *Law & Order* do DAs follow a death back to people at the corporate or other remote levels who might be held responsible. Life ought to imitate art in this instance—doing so might save a few lives.

There was absolutely no publicity whatsoever about the handyman's death case. I didn't mind its absence, even if I thought OCME did deserve some pats on the back for solving it and saving the lives of future tenants who might have been accidentally electrocuted. At the end of the day, that's our job, one of the many ways in which we work to preserve public health.

Preserving public safety is an often-overlooked component of what we do at the OCME. Indeed, most people are unaware that many public-health safety innovations and breakthrough research emerge from information collected from death investigators. The OCME participates in the Medical Examiner and Coroner Alert Program (MECAP), a national program that informs authorities and manufacturers about product and therapy safety matters. Many of the safety devices and innovations used every day all over the world—seatbelts, bicycle helmets, child-proof pill bottles, warning labels on toys that contain choking hazards—come in part or in whole from the work of MEs and coroners all across the United States who collect information after a tragedy to help prevent a similar one from occurring. This program has had some great successes—like prodding manufacturers of electronically operated garage doors to install a safety device that prevents those doors from slamming down unexpectedly and killing people, and similar devices to stop car windows from closing when they meet resistance, so as not to garrote a child. Like making certain that the slats on a baby crib are close enough together so that they cannot catch a baby's head in them and strangle the baby to death. Like lobbying to make smoke and carbon monoxide detectors mandatory equipment in multifamily dwellings.

New York City is big—really big. One way to fathom just how huge this sprawling metropolis is comes from having intimate contact with its hundreds of miles of train tracks. New York's subway system is so vast that it contains nearly as many stations as all the other subway systems in the country combined. During an average workday in the city, more than twelve million people will be hurrying about, each seemingly intent on getting where they need to go and not paying very much attention to what's going on around them or who might be in their way. The wonder is not that we have traffic and pedestrian fatalities but that we don't have more than we do.

New York is also a destination city; more than forty million visitors each year come through the Big Apple, and, statistically, if you get that many visitors, some of them are going to die. Some tourists even *arrive* dead.

I've had to investigate transportation-related deaths of every variety, including those of pedestrians, bicyclists, and of course riders in planes, trains, and automobiles—not to mention boats. With the exception of the Bronx, all of New York City is located on islands, and we have quite a number of docks, piers, and shipyards; many major cruise liners regularly visit the city. The city's labyrinthine transportation system has been the scene of some strange deaths. And the stranger they were, during my years as a supervising MLI, the greater the likelihood that I would be the one called to the scene.

My least favorite deaths are those in the subway. I've always hated New York's subways, probably because I lived for four years in Montreal and there saw what a subway system should be like. By comparison, New York's system is simply abysmal. I am told that it has gotten better since the late 1970s and 1980s, when I rode it to and from school and referred to it as the world's longest urinal. I stopped taking the subway around the time I graduated from PA school and vowed never to ride it again. Busses work just as well, and they don't smell as bad. Fortunately, in my job at OCME, I had a car to take me around the city, so just about the only times I went down into the subway was when someone was hit by a train.

Something about the death of a person struck by a train captures the very root of horror in our imaginations. Among the earliest film footage ever shot was that of a helpless woman bound to the tracks, while nearby the evil villain with the unbelievably long, waxed mustache chortled and gleefully rubbed his hands together. In current movies as well as in the silent film era, the damsel in distress is inevitably rescued in the nick of time by the hero—who must have been resting in the makeup trailer during the cases I was called on to investigate. In reality, instead of being bound to the tracks, the victim in most subway deaths falls or is pushed off the platform and is unable to get out of the way of the oncoming train. It is every commuter's worst nightmare.

One of the most horrible such deaths I've ever had to deal with was that of a young female visitor to the city who was pushed off a subway platform by a deranged homeless man into the path of an onrushing subway train. Her body was burned by the third rail and crushed by the train—charred and mangled beyond belief, indeed beyond recognition as human and female. Detectives at the scene assured me that witnesses stated that the victim was a woman, but when I examined the remains at the scene, the only way I could tell that she had been a woman was by some long hair and scraps of her underwear. Seeing her mutilated body on the tracks is one of the awful pictures that I carry in my head. It haunts me to this day.

The case received a tremendous amount of media attention, perhaps because the victim had been a vibrant, beautiful young woman with a promising life ahead of her. She had come to New York to seek her fortune and instead had met an awful end. She personified for me all the horror of sudden, terrible death in the subway. As I said, I hate the subway.

One of the scariest places I've ever been was a subway side tunnel, off the main track and seldom used. It was seventy feet below street level, dark, damp, and infested with vermin, garbage, and every other kind of filth. We'd been called to the scene because a routine maintenance crew, in checking the area, had noticed a foul stench, followed their noses, and found a body. (That must have been fun.) When I was given the call sheet for the case, I had been somewhat amused by the cops' report of "decomposed man, struck by train," which had made me imagine a dead and decomposed man walking like a zombie along the tracks until he was struck by a train. Actually, a poor derelict who was making his home in one of the innumerable unused tunnels deep in the subway system had been hit by a passing train, and had been knocked into a side tunnel, where he died, perhaps a month before he was found. The exact PMI was hard to determine because rats had been feasting on him.

While trains do kill people, it is rare that one arrives in the city with a dead body *aboard*. This is not so with planes and boats. The most interesting, non-crash-related plane death our office ever handled involved a dead woman in the seat of an airplane that had recently landed at JFK Airport from the Caribbean island of Jamaica. The decedent was a little old woman in a floppy hat, and she was so advanced into rigor mortis that it was difficult to remove her from her seat. Which raised the obvious question: How long had she been dead? The plane trip from Jamaica took five hours, and full rigor usually requires about twelve hours to set in.

By the time we arrived on the scene, the plane was empty except for a few crew members, the police, the dead passenger, still in her seat in the rear of the plane, and her equally elderly husband, who sat quietly in the first-class cabin where he had been asked to wait. In an interview, he told us a simple but extraordinary story.

That morning, the last day of their trip to Jamaica, he had awoken in a hotel room to find that his beloved wife of more than fifty years had died in her sleep. He sat on the bed with her for quite a while, trying to decide what to do. The couple was not well off financially, but had saved for a long time to take this trip to the Caribbean. The husband reasoned (correctly) that it would cost many thousands of dollars to have a funeral home prepare and ship his wife's body back home. But it dawned on him that he had a perfectly good return ticket for her for the flight to New York that was leaving in a few hours. He dressed his wife, and asked the front desk of the hotel to send up a porter with a wheelchair. He dispatched the luggage with the porter, and in the meantime somehow sandwiched her into that wheelchair and took her down to the lobby. Still in the wheelchair, she rode to the airport in a van, her face hidden by the large floppy hat. At the gate, he asked for and received special help in preboarding his "sick" wife who was "sedated and napping." Helpful flight attendants eased her gently into her seat. (Full rigor had still not set in.) Had his plane not been delayed a few hours in take off, he might have gotten away with the whole deal. But the plane was delayed, so when they finally touched down in New York, she had been dead for so many hours that she was in full rigor mortis, and the napping story had worn a little thin.

Further investigation revealed that the elderly woman had a history of congestive heart failure and had indeed died of natural causes; OCME issued a death certificate for her and released her body to the husband on the condition that he hire a funeral home to prepare and bury her. Although he must have broken a dozen laws in bringing her to New York, he was not charged or prosecuted for the stunt. To be quite frank, we all admired his moxie.

New York City sees deaths from car crashes, perhaps not as often as interstate highways do, but often enough, and plenty of pedestrian deaths. More often than not, a pedestrian death happens when a person who took a step or two off the curb into a street as he or she was waiting for a traffic light to change is struck by a truck turning a corner, hitting the person with its back wheels.

Another type of victim that we see often in the autopsy room is the bicycle messenger. A fixture in Manhattan, these kamikazes on two wheels constantly dart in and out of traffic. Almost every driver, after seeing these bicyclists weave between thundering trucks, buses, and maniacal cabbies, has been known to exclaim, "They must get killed all the time doing that." Indeed they do—regularly. It's almost enough to make you want to use the subway.

Given the volume of traffic-related deaths such as bike messengers, you would presume that OCME would be called to a traffic-related scene investigation every day, but we actually respond to very few. New York City does not allow us to investigate vehicular deaths (traffic accidents) as thoroughly as our counterparts upstate or on Long Island look into deaths on, say, an interstate highway. In this big city, there's a sense that traffic must be kept moving, that we cannot cordon off the scene for too long, or else we'll cause gridlock. Accordingly, the OCME is not called to every fatal traffic accident scene; a police department unit, the Accident Investigation Squad, handles most of these.

This is logical, except that vehicular homicide is one of the easiest forms of murder to get away with. "Oh, no, I didn't mean to run over her; it was an accident." Sure, the police department accident investigation teams are good, but they are not as well trained in medical matters as OCME people are, and it stands to reason that since OCME is charged with the responsibility of determining the manner of death, ascertaining it in vehicular deaths should be our responsibility—but it's not.

If you're going to die aboard a ship—and people do die while on cruises, all the time—the *Queen Elizabeth II* has the nicest little ocean-going morgue in which I've ever had tea.

Most cruise liners have some form of morgue, and many of these are state of the art. The passengers on cruises tend to be middle-aged and older; they dance, exercise, and put themselves through all sorts of unaccustomed exertions after they've feasted on food and liquor. On any self-respecting cruise ship, eating is the single greatest form of activity; the high-fat, high-cholesterol smorgasbord is in action, 24/7. After three or four days of this sort of gluttony, combined with unaccustomed exertion, the potential for guests having either a stroke or a heart attack is high. Though I suppose there are far worse ways and times to die.

Big cruise ships always have a doctor on board, and an infirmary, so why shouldn't we expect that such a ship would also contain a small, tastefully appointed, refrigerated morgue that is not, by the way, connected to the refrigerators in which the ship carries its food? I know that cruise lines don't go out of their way to include such information in their advertising packets, but in truth, cruise ships are floating cities, and actuaries will tell you that if a large number of people are together in one location, particularly if many of them are of a "certain" age, some will die. And the likelihood of someone keeling over while aboard is raised by all that unusual stress that I mentioned. Accurate statistics on how many people die a year aboard cruise ships are very hard to come by, for reasons that you can easily imagine, but between natural deaths, accidents, suicides, and homicides, the per capita death rate on board a large ship is probably no different than that of a major city. We at OCME are regularly called to the docks along Manhattan's West Side to meet the cruise ships when they arrive with a "special" passenger or two.

That dead passenger may be on board because no other jurisdiction was willing to deal with him or her. Gone are the days when people who died at sea were tossed over the side to sleep with the fishes. Deaths that occur at sea are supposed to be off-loaded from the ship at the next port of call, but frequently they aren't, because in many ports of call the authorities don't choose to deal with dead people from another jurisdiction and refuse to have the body off-loaded in their port. That is why some of those who die while on cruise ships end up in the port of New York—where on principle we will not refuse to examine a dead person, no matter where he or she came from.

Here's the drill: When the ship arrives, we are summoned to dockside, usually very early in the morning. Often the report of the death has arrived at OCME in the middle of the night, long before the ship docks. It has been radioed by the crew to the harbormaster, and then on to us so that we can be standing by when the ship docks. The passengers will want to get off and go home, but if there is a death aboard, technically, they can't disembark, at least not until OCME says they can. It is within our power to quarantine the whole ship and to not let anyone off if we suspect that the death was caused by a communicable disease. This painful possibility is why we are treated very nicely when we arrive; we are generally met at the pier by a ship's officer and escorted to the infirmary and the mini-morgue, where we meet with the ship's doctor and perhaps with the family of the deceased. On many occasions, the offer has been made to me of a cup of tea—or other refreshments—to be served after all the "pesky paperwork" is done, in the hope that I will do my work quickly and the live passengers will not be bothered with having to stay aboard a second longer than they want to.

If we did suspect a death was due to a contagious disease and had to send the body for an autopsy, the passengers could be forced to remain aboard until we ascertained the exact cause of death and determined whether releasing the passengers posed a danger to the public health. Fortunately, I've never had to send a body from a ship to be autopsied. I shudder to think of the chaos that would ensue if I had to quarantine a cruise ship. The natural deaths that I have seen were all of the variety I described earlier, usually attributable to overeating and overexertion in older folks with underlying disease factors. The onboard investigation is usually limited to interviewing the ship's doctor and the family and taking a quick look at the body before releasing it to the family, who usually has a funeral director (also alerted by the ship long before it arrived) with a hearse standing by at the dock.

We do, of course, issue death certificates for such bodies, even though the death occurred outside of New York City. There is no other choice—the cruise ship can't do it. Those certificates are a bit unusual in that they note the exact latitude and longitude at which the death occurred. This archaic practice tickles me, but really, there is no other way to describe the location of the death. In the ocean, there are no street addresses.

Of all the investigations I've done in which a body arrived dead to New York City, one revealed to me that some people really do have actual skeletons in their closets. In what became one of my more memorable cases, I was summoned to a most unusual clothing store in which human remains had been found. The store was actually a large apartment in an Upper West Side pre–World War II building—the kind of apartment that has fourteen-foot-high ceilings and a seemingly endless number of rooms—and the shop specialized in transvestite clothing and costumes. The owner of the store, the sole occupant of the apartment, was a cross-dresser who ran "her" shop out of four of the apartment's twelve rooms. Before going to the scene, I received this information over the phone from a detective who also told me that the owner had recently died, but that it was not *her* death that I would be investigating.

According to the detective, the storeowner had evidently been beloved in the cross-dressing world for providing the very best in women's clothes for men. After her death, some of her friends had gotten together and thrown a party and rummage sale at the shop to raise money for her funeral. During the sale, a mummified body had been found in a closet.

When I arrived on the scene, I learned that the finder of the remains had been poking around in the back of a very large walk-in closet and, on a top shelf, had found a surprisingly heavy valise at which he tugged until it came crashing down. The determined shopper, I was informed, was an off-duty NYPD detective, who had been at the rummage sale in search of a costume for the upcoming Halloween parade in Manhattan's Greenwich Village. Prying open the locked valise, the detective had found it filled with a large black plastic garbage bag. He also noticed a certain musty aroma, which, I am sure, must have worried him. He opened the bag and found yet another plastic garbage bag inside of it. Abandoning the gentle approach, he ripped open a hole in a corner of the four bags covering the contents, and revealed a dried and shriveled human hand. Peeking through the hole, he discerned the mummified remains of a human being.

For the detective, finding these remains must have initially presented a dilemma, I mused, because making a report of this mummified person might well mean that he'd have to tell his superiors his reason for being in the shop in the first place. But this didn't stop him for very long, if at all, because he did his duty.

Arriving at the scene, I realized that the off-duty detective had done a great job of securing it, because the valise was still in the closet. A uniformed cop and a couple of squad detectives watched me with no attempt to hide their amusement as I pushed my way through racks of long pink boas, neon-colored sequined evening gowns, piles of very large ladies' shoes, wigs of every imaginable style and color, and stacks of garments that my grandmother would have referred to as unmentionables.

Kneeling on the floor amid the surreal contents of that closet, I very carefully opened the valise and removed a little bit more of the wrappings, just enough to verify that they did indeed enfold the remains of a human being. I tried to disturb the suitcase and its contents as little as possible, because when dealing with any body packaged in wrappings, it's always best to wait for full examination in the autopsy room. Less evidence is lost if the body and its wrappings are examined there. But before I closed the suitcase, I noticed two clues that suggested we were dealing with a death that was quite a few years old.

Newspapers wrapped around the body dated from the 1970s. And there was a soda-can tab of a type I had not seen in a long time (a metal ring attached to a sort of little metal tongue, a tab that was designed to be pulled completely off the can). Years ago, antilittering legislation had forced manufacturers to stop using that type of tab.

The next morning, X-rays of the suitcase showed us a body curled into the fetal position, wrapped in layers as though the suitcase was a macabre womb, with a bullet inside the skull that told us we were dealing with a homicide even before we opened the suitcase itself. The autopsy on the mummified remains revealed that the decedent was a man who had been killed by a single gunshot wound to the head from a small-caliber weapon and the bullet was still lodged in his mummified brain. The victim had been short and very slender—the perfect body type to have ended up as a mummy.

The newspapers and soda tab, combined with the extreme mummification of the body, indicated that the body had probably been in the suitcase for more than twenty years. Even so, we were able to successfully identify the body by fingerprinting the mummy. However,

133

as you might imagine, obtaining those prints was a challenge. Well-preserved skin is so dry that attempting to "ink" the fingers and roll them for prints will result in unreadable blotches. Instead, over the years OCME experts have developed an ingenious method for obtaining fingerprints from mummies, one that most people, even at OCME, find rather icky to watch. First a syringe injects saline into the leather-like skin of the mummy's hands to rehydrate and soften the tissue. Once the skin is again pliable, we ever so carefully peel it off the hands, beginning at the wrists, and continuing down to the fingertips. A good peel results in a perfect inside-out glove of human skin that can then be further softened if necessary by soaking it in a saline bath. When the skin is finally ready, an examiner dons a tight-fitting latex glove over which the human skin is carefully rolled, reversing the peeling process by which it was removed. If done correctly, the examiner now wears the skin of a dead man on his hand, and, wearing this gruesome glove, he inks "his" fingers and rolls them onto the print card, leaving the prints of the dead guy.

The excellent prints we obtained were then circulated around the country, and specifically to the Midwestern city from which the newspapers in the suitcase had come. By matching his prints, authorities there were able to identify the mummified remains as those of a burglar with an extensive rap sheet who had gone missing in the mid-1970s. As best we could reconstruct the story, he had tried to rob the transvestite store owner's previous shop, located in that city, and had been shot dead in the course of the robbery. Perhaps fearing that she would be prosecuted for the shooting, she never reported the incident and, instead, wrapped her dead burglar in newspaper and plastic bags, stuffed his body into a suitcase, and hid him in a closet. And during the ensuing decades, she took along her skeleton in the closet whenever and wherever she moved.

Eventually, the family of the long-deceased burglar showed up in New York, claimed the body of their dead relative, and took him home for burial.

NINE

I CAN NO longer remember every one of the more than eight thousand deaths that I have investigated, although a photo of a particular death scene can sometimes bring back memories of that particular dead body. On occasion, even looking at a photo doesn't summon up the memories and reviewing the case file makes me feel that I'm reading someone else's notes or summary. However, hundreds of my cases have been so memorable that I have no chance of forgetting them.

Each of those is indelibly imprinted on my mind—some are memorable for their "Agatha Christie" moments, while others are unforgettable for different reasons. High on my list of Agatha Christie moments was arriving at an upscale apartment in one of Manhattan's swankiest neighborhoods on a weekend evening and making my way through the vestiges of a recently concluded seventieth birthday party toward a den/office at the end of a hall. I saw inside that room a man slumped forward over his desk, facing away from the door, in a chair on the visitor's side of the desk. I was told that this was the birthday boy, a well-regarded financial professional—dead at his own party. Tilting him back in the chair, I discovered a letter opener thrust into his chest and, from the looks of it, right into his heart.

This could have been murder; someone could have come up from behind him and stabbed him in the chest. But it was equally possible that his death had been a suicide. Although a layperson might think that a would-be suicide couldn't stab himself to death in the chest, I know differently. I've even seen one man who stabbed himself *multiple* times in the chest until he got it right.

The relatives of the man lying dead at his desk said he had a history of psychiatric problems but that these had not seemed very serious. I checked some of the medications and hospital paperwork in the room and had to agree with that estimate. Adding to the mystery was that I couldn't find a suicide note. The letter opener was nowhere near as sharp as a kitchen knife, and it would have required tremendous force to push it through the man's body into the heart. Could he have done it himself, without aid? I was dubious, yet there was no indication that anyone else had been involved in the death. The den was immaculate, with no indications of any struggle. There were several delicate figurines on the desk that surely would have been smashed in a tussle. Aside from the wound caused by the letter opener sticking out of his chest, the victim displayed no other surface damage.

Given the suspicious nature of this death, it was imperative that I bring him in for an autopsy, which caused some difficulties for the Jewish family. Since it was in the evening, we would not be able to perform the autopsy and have the body ready for burial within twenty-four hours as Jewish law demanded, but I promised the family that we'd do it as quickly as possible so that they could have a proper funeral. The autopsy confirmed that the decedent had, indeed, died of a single stab wound to the heart and that there was no sign of a struggle. The angle at which the letter opener had gone in was consistent with his having used his own hand, so suicide was still a possibility. However, in New York City, to label a death as a suicide, we need an additional piece of information not required for any other manner of death. We must prove, of course, that the person did the act themselves, but moreover we must be able to prove *intent*—to aver that by this action the victim has deliberately taken his or her own life. This requirement is common sense since, in a suicide, intent *makes* the manner of death. In this particular death, even though we were confident it was not a homicide, and it was unlikely that the letter opener ended up in the victim's chest by accident, we had no way of proving intent. No way of asserting categorically that the decedent did this to himself and meant to take his own life by this action. We certainly could not do so by the next day when we released the body for its funeral. So we issued a death certificate that read "pending further investigation," and continued investigating. As the family was preparing for the burial, a relative found—in a bag containing the dead man's *tallis*, his ceremonial prayer shawl worn for religious observances—a suicide note. He had been depressed, and the final straw had been that he felt that the guest list for his birthday party did not contain enough distinguished names. He had placed the suicide note in a location where he knew it would eventually be found because Jewish men are buried in their prayer shawls. Holographic examination of the note revealed that it was authentic and in the victim's handwriting, so the case was closed. The manner of death was listed as suicide.

The actual reason that this man committed suicide was not, of course, a guest list; the real reason for the suicide was also in his note—pain. He was in pain, mental pain, and possibly even associated physical pain. That was consistent with every other suicide note I'd seen—and I've seen more than enough of them. They all mention pain, unbearable pain.

What I have come to understand, from years of investigating such deaths, and what I am convinced families, friends, and doctors of would-be suicides must understand, is that the pain is there, and it is very real. Pain cannot be dismissed as "only mental," and, indeed, it often consists of physical pain accompanied by, and worsened by, mental anguish. In the suicide's own words, and in the words of their loved ones left behind (whom I frequently have to interview), the victim is always described as being in unbearable torment. Given the lengths that some people go to kill themselves, the wish to escape that torment is the motivating factor for the suicide that makes the most sense to me. Many suicides conveyed in their notes that they were being burned alive by pain that no one else could see, and they felt that killing themselves was the only way to stop the agony.

In cultures different from the United States, suicide is not considered a failure of the courage to face life, but as a legitimate response to certain life situations. In Japan for example, suicide is highly ritualized and one who commits suicide is respected, particularly if the deed is done in a spectacular manner. Immigrants to our shores from such cultures sometimes do things we might not comprehend at first glance, but when we view the act within its cultural context we have a better chance of understanding the motivation—intent—of the victim. Case in point was the suicide of a Japanese nanny. I was called to a death scene in another, even more posh, Manhattan apartment, where two young children were in near hysteria because their Japanese nanny lay dead in front of them, with a sharp kitchen knife through her gut. Her other hand clutched a spatula.

The story, as I reconstructed it from conversations with neighbors and with the children, was this: The apartment belonged to a wealthy couple who were not at home at the time. They had left the youngsters in the care of the nanny, who had been with the family for some time.

However, the nanny had been having a difficult time controlling the children. When they wouldn't obey her, she lost face and threatened the children with committing seppuku (ritual suicide) right in front of them to shame them. Being very young and American, the kids had no idea what she was talking about, but she persisted on this line, and they persisted in disobeying her orders. So she went into the kitchen and seized the knife and the spatula. I never found out why she wielded the spatula, but I wondered if it had been used to try to spank one of the children. In any event, she used the knife to perform her ritual suicide right in front of the children.

Investigating this case, I learned that in Japan ritual suicide has more to do with honor than with pain, but to my American eyes the mental rationale in this case made even less sense to me than the case of the suicide at the birthday party.

There is one type of suicide that I fully understand and wholeheartedly condone. I believe that terminally ill patients with intractable disease should have the right, by law, to end their lives comfortably and with dignity. During the mid-1990s, we saw a fair number of suicides that were right out of the book *Final Exit*, an unfortunate bestseller by Derek Humphry, founder of the Hemlock Society. I say unfortunate because his book is really a textbook that shows people the various ways to commit suicide. On a disconcertingly regular basis, I would find people dead in their dwelling places, with a copy of the book nearby, having used one of the book's well-described methods to end their lives. Many of those people had been dying of a terminal illness, and for them, I suppose, Humphry's book was a blessing. But not all the *Final Exit* suicides were of terminal patients, and that is the part that bothers me.

All over the country, mayors and police commissioners talk a lot about the homicide rate (and they should), but city governmental officials almost never mention the suicide rate, which in New York hovers just under one thousand a year (and we should all be talking about that). Currently, almost twice as many people commit suicide as are being murdered. I have wondered how many of those who commit suicide might have been able to live on, with better lives, had they received proper counseling and medication? It is impossible to give a numerical answer, but my guess is that at least some of them would have had some of their problems ameliorated, and would have been encouraged to go on living.

A vast majority of people die of natural causes and in New York City, as elsewhere in the United States, most people die in hospitals. It makes more sense here, perhaps, because we sure do have a lot of hospitals—in fact, more hospital beds than there are in most small countries. And it's not only New Yorkers who utilize them. The concomitant of having many available beds and good medical care is something that we at OCME recognized a long time ago: New York is a tourist destination not only for its theaters, restaurants, museums, and night life but also for its spectacular medical care, provided by some of the very best health care facilities in the world, including the sharpest of cutting-edge therapy. Yes, medical tourism swells the ranks of our sick and increases the number of deaths reported every year to our office. We at OCME don't discriminate on the basis of where you're from originally or even recently; all we care about is whether you've died in our jurisdiction. If so, we'll look into your death as though you were a born-in-the-Bronx, died-in-Brooklyn, "Noo Yawkuh."

According to the most recent annual summary of New York City's Department of Vital Statistics, approximately 60 percent of deaths in New York City occur in a medical facility. In almost every such instance, the medical-facility deaths that require OCME's attention are simply called in to us and handled over the phone by an MLI in collaboration with the reporting doctor. But in certain instances in which people die in hospitals, a scene visit is required—usually for a very good reason. Some of these I remember very clearly.

In one city hospital, a homeless man who was wandering around late one night found the deserted rehabilitation department and decided that a physical therapy tub looked like a great place to take a bath. I guess he wasn't used to bathing because he managed to drown in the tub. Actually, the tub was pretty deep, about five feet, with steep, slick metal sides. At another hospital, one of the regular floor nurses blew her brains out with a large-caliber revolver, and did so in a public bathroom on the ground floor of the hospital, for reasons that never became clear to us.

Oddly enough, one particular hospital kept having deaths that were recorded on video. One patient with a psychiatric history committed suicide by throwing himself from a fourteenth-floor interior stairwell; though the initial jump was not recorded, each floor's security camera recorded his descent, all the way to impact. We were able to put together an eerie still-frame montage of his final seconds.

Even stranger was the videotape of a death in that hospital's sleep-disorder clinic. A female patient came in for evaluation in the hospital's special lab, where attendants hooked her up to various electronic monitors while she lay in a comfortable-looking bed and tried to sleep. In an adjacent control room her heart rate, breathing, and oxygen levels were being monitored by attendants who also could watch her every toss and turn on multiple video cameras. But at one point during this diagnostic procedure, she had a seizure—her susceptibility to seizures was one reason why she was being studied—and in the midst of that seizure, she rolled over in bed so that she was on her stomach, facedown in her pillow. The lone attendant was on break, and thus did not know that the unconscious patient, in a postseizure state, was unable to lift her face off the pillow. She smothered to death.

Later, at OCME, as we watched the video of her death, which took an excruciating half hour, I kept fighting the urge to run into the lab and rescue her. Because of the immediacy of videotape, it was difficult to keep in mind that the images we were seeing had been recorded the day before. The camera's perspective, looking through the glass into her room, gave you the feeling that you were right there in the lab and that all you had to do to save her was run into her room and turn her over. Had someone been watching her during that half hour, or at least been attending to the monitors, he or she would have done just that—gone in and turned her over, because they would have seen what we eventually saw, a day late and a life short. An attendant would have heard monitor alarms go off as her heart rate dropped, her breathing slowed, and her blood oxygen fell.

It was inexplicable to me that the monitoring technician had simply not been present while the patient slowly died, but supposedly he was on a legitimate break with no one there to cover for him during that period. We ruled that death to have been an accident. Shouldn't there have been a finding of criminal negligence? That was not the business of the OCME; such findings can only be made by the DA's office and are usually only made when the negligent person was in the process of doing something illegal. If the technician in attendance at the sleep study had been out of the room buying drugs, or engaged in some other activity that was illegal, then a case might have been made. But since he was on a scheduled break, he could not be held criminally responsible for the death. Which isn't to say that the hospital should not have been held *civilly* liable for it. But civil liability is no more OCME's purview than is criminal liability. I don't know if the family sued the hospital, but I hope they did.

One of the ugliest deaths I encountered during a scene investigation at a hospital was that of a patient who died when the gurney on which he was strapped was sliced in two by a malfunctioning elevator. The OCME headquarters is located in an area of Manhattan known informally as Bedpan Alley because of the large number of hospitals in close proximity to one another. This death occurred at one of these close-by hospitals, and, in my rush to get to the scene, I simply ran out of my office in my shirtsleeves, leaving behind my OCME photo ID and my badge.

At the hospital, there was near-chaos, including a quite frantic Latino family of the victim, the bloody elevator scene itself, and an apoplectic hospital administrator. I tried to enter the scene, but without an ID, I was stopped by hospital personnel; however, the cops who had responded to the emergency call knew me and let me through. I examined the bloody elevator and the victim. An orderly had been in the midst of pushing the patient strapped to the gurney into the elevator. Somehow, with the elevator's doors open and the gurney half in and half out, the elevator began to descend, crushing the gurney and just about tearing the patient in half. After I examined the scene, I then wanted to speak with the decedent's family. They were still talking to the beleaguered hospital administrator, and when I walked over and introduced myself, I guess this was more than he could handle. He actually began to gibber (I had never seen anyone do that before) and demanded to see my ID. I groaned to myself and ruefully admitted I didn't have it on me. This was a day when the administrator must have felt that nothing was in his control, but here was one thing he could: an insistent outsider with no ID. He immediately attempted to evict me and forbid me from talking to the family.

I explained to him, calmly, one more time, that I was from the ME's office and I'd simply left my ID at my desk. Regardless, he had security throw me out of the hospital.

I marched back in, escorted this time by the police who knew me, and who vouched for my identity and for the fact that the ME's office has the duty of examining the death scene and the victim and of speaking with the family. However, the blustery administrator—worried, no doubt, about a potential lawsuit against the hospital for negligence— still refused to let me talk to the family. It wasn't rational, but he wasn't in a thinking frame of mind. The police kindly offered to intercede for me.

I told them it wasn't necessary; push did not have to come to shove since I had already examined the scene of the death to my satisfaction. So I told the administrator that I would talk to the family outside the hospital if he wouldn't let me speak with them inside and, over his shoulder, issued an invitation to the family to join me on the sidewalk. They did, and we spoke for a few moments. I explained what the next steps would be and that I would see them again tomorrow at OCME headquarters.

Needless to say, I never thereafter left the OCME to go to a scene without my ID in my pocket.

The elevator death was an accident, but other deaths in hospitals are not so accidental. Through my work at OCME, I became, unwillingly, an expert on the various ways in which a patient could get himself or herself killed while in a hospital and on just which hospitals were killing what sorts of patients, and how often. This became sought-after information.

Just as at Thanksgiving, because of my expertise, I was always asked to carve the turkey, I was also asked in less festive settings to be a physician/hospital rating service. A friend, before undergoing surgery, would call and say, "I'm going in to Such-and-Such Hospital and Dr. So-and-So is gonna take out my whatsit." Then the friend might couch a question such as, "Is the surgeon any good?" or "Is the hospital a good one?" but what he or she was actually asking me was, "Has this doctor slaughtered any patients recently?" and "Does this hospital regularly report disastrous outcomes to OCME?" I always gave answers that incorporated the best of my knowledge, but even when my recommendations were sterling, I knew that my friends had, and still have, good reason to worry when they enter a hospital—any hospital.

Hospitals are very dangerous places. Between overtired residents, overworked nurses, understaffed wards, complicated machinery, drugs that can have sledgehammer side effects, and good old-fashioned human error, the modern hospital has more ways to kill you than did the Spanish Inquisition. Some of those proved frightening, even to this seasoned investigator.

In one instance, a young athlete went into a hospital for a routine elective surgery and never came out. Exercise had bulked up his arm muscles to the point that they were causing pressure on the nerves running through his elbow, giving him a continuous sensation of the sort that happens to all of us when we hit our "funny bone." He was admitted to the hospital for a standard operation that would relieve this pressure. It was performed, but in the recovery room, the otherwise perfectly healthy patient developed postoperative hypertension, a not-all-that-uncommon side effect of anesthesia. Then—and unfortunately for the patient—an intern became rambunctious. The patient's blood pressure was climbing fast, and the intern called down to the pharmacy for Esmolol (a rarely used but very potent beta-blocker) to relieve this high blood pressure. The rookie intern, greener than the scrubs he was wearing but possessing a cowboy attitude not yet tempered by the life he was about to take, then made a dosing mistake of massive proportions. The young intern mistakenly administered, instead of a small dosage, the entire bottle of the beta-blocker, via a "pushing" intravenous method. Having never before used this extremely powerful drug, the intern was unaware that the large bottle the pharmacy had sent up contained enough of the medication for a twenty-four-hour drip. (The pharmacy sent that because it did not carry the smaller, single-dose ampoule.) Before all the dosage had been pushed into the athelete's system, he went into irreversible asystole (flatline) and died.

Word quickly went around the hospital that the intern had "boxed" a patient—that is, killed him. The case was reported to OCME, where it was ruled an accident. Had the intern been a licensed physician at the time, his license to practice medicine might have been taken from him. Since he was not yet licensed and because he was acting under the supervision of more experienced physicians, the authorities could take no action against the intern. The only punishment he received was a suspension from the hospital for a minor amount of time.

When things go wrong in hospitals, they can go horribly wrong. In another case at the same hospital, a death occurred in the ICU when a resident physician neglected to deflate a balloon at the end of a catheter before removing the catheter from the patient's subclavian artery. This particular catheter, called a Swan-Ganz, is put into critically ill patients to closely monitor their cardiovascular functions. The balloon at the tip of the catheter holds it in place inside the artery right near the heart, and this balloon must be deflated before the catheter is removed from the artery. In this instance, it wasn't, and when the catheter was pulled the inflated balloon burst the artery. The patient bled to death in a few seconds. This same hospital had a third similar death when a guide wire inserted in an artery for a similar procedure was not properly taken out.

These cases bring up the larger question of the efficacy of all therapy. One of my tenets is that eventually all therapy fails, which I can prove since no one gets out of this life alive. Moreover, most hospital deaths are not the result of egregious error but of the normal progress of pathology. However, modern therapy can mask the natural progression of disease. So quite often, when we are evaluating what has happened in a hospital bed or in the ER, the questions arise: Did the underlying disease assert itself, or did the patient actually die from complications of the therapy? Or at some point did applying proper treatment slip over into accidentally killing the patient? Cases involving these matters are absolutely among the most difficult presented to OCME. Often the decision is a judgment call based on the nuances of a particular set of circumstances.

The tenet that all therapy fails has as a corollary the notion that death can be a *positive* outcome of a hospital stay. By this I mean that death is a natural occurrence, and in every human instance, it is an eventual one, so that sometimes a death in the hospital is inevitable and thus a proper outcome. This is not the view that is taught to medical students and residents, who have drilled into them the idea that death is the enemy, that they must fight decay and disease all the time and at all costs. Obeying this "always fight off death" edict sometimes causes physicians to make a mockery of the basic commandment of the Hippocratic oath, "First, do no harm," by keeping a patient alive when the more natural course of events—the more natural outcome of the progress of his or her disease or condition—is a natural death. Sometimes patients are kept alive by such extreme artificial measures that when they die, it becomes almost impossible to sort out the original

145

underlying natural disease, which disappears under a welter of thera-peutic complications.

This understanding of excessive and sometimes wrong-headed treatment plays a large role when I speak to people about the care they receive in a hospital or doctor's office. Many people seem to believe that when they're admitted to a hospital they must surrender their rights and freedom of choice when it comes to their therapy. It is vital for patients to realize that everyone—whether in a hospital or a doc-tor's office—has the right to (and should) double-check every dosage of medicine they receive. In addition, the patient has the right to find out who is about to do that invasive procedure on them and question that person's ability to handle such a procedure. Has that person done it before? If it is a relatively junior person, is he or she under close su-pervision while doing it? If the patient does not deem the answers given to be satisfactory, he or she should refuse consent to the proce-dure until the patient has obtained answers that allow him or her to believe that the procedure will be done properly. I am also an advocate of writing up a health care proxy—a patient designating someone to legally make medical decisions for him or her if the patient is incapac-itated—and having it handy, to prevent ending up as a guinea pig in some doctor's experiment.

When things do go wrong at hospitals, families routinely request that the ME's office do autopsies on deaths that they believe are suspi-cious, and they ask us such questions as, "How do you know the hospi-tals isn't lying about the cause and manner of death?" and, "Could they be covering up a mistake?"

When I'm asked such questions, my answer is this: nothing pre-vents hospitals from writing up a death as though it were a nonerror—except that the hospitals know that by and large they wouldn't be able to get away with it. To hide such an error would require a massive con-spiracy involving all of the forty to fifty people who had been in touch with the patient in the hospital, risking the probability that among them there would be one or two who would not go along or who would blab the truth to family, the police, or the decedent's insurance com-pany investigators. Also, any autopsy by our office would likely uncover any falsity. Therefore, hospitals mostly do not lie about these deaths, although now and then I have run across individuals who fudge a little.

After all, some things in the dying process are susceptible to multiple interpretations. Did the patient expire from the complications of the disease—that is, a natural death—or because some therapy failed? Sometimes it's six of one, half a dozen of another. For the most part, I saw very little effort by hospitals to deliberately avoid reporting deaths properly. Those hospital personnel who have the responsibility of overseeing the reporting of deaths don't have MD licenses; they are clerks and administrators, which means they would not lose their licenses should the death be ruled the fault of the doctor. As a result, they have no reason to be complicit in a hospital cover-up and are quite straightforward with us. Moreover, hospitals and physicians are insured to cover complications of therapy.

If a case is not reported to us when it should be, the usual reason is ignorance of the statutes. However, once in a while some doctor naively tries to cover something up by writing a creative death certificate—and not always to conceal a deliberate fraud. I once had a case in which a young doctor at a county hospital issued a death certificate that read "Cardiopulmonary Arrest" (CPA) as the cause of death. I decided to call the doctor. At first she did not want to discuss the case with me, but after one of the senior hospital administrators explained to her that she was required by law to answer my questions, she acquiesced. From my questions, I learned that the decedent had committed suicide. He was from a devout Catholic family, and the doctor, still an intern, was simply trying to heed the family's plea to certify the death as "natural" so that no stigma would be associated with the death, and the Catholic cemetery (which might not allow a suicide to be buried in consecrated ground) would bury him as the family wished.

Had the doctor known how to properly make out the death certificate, she might have gotten away with this fraud. But as with most of the physicians with whom I interacted, she had no idea how to actually write up a cause of death, fill out a death certificate, or even properly make the diagnosis of death. Now I am not talking about verifying that the decedent is in fact no longer among the living; even the greenest intern is able to recognize a flatline on an EKG machine. I am talking about the *diagnosis,* that is to say, the circumstances and cause that led to the person's death. The ability to make this "final diagnosis" is something that is not taught in medical school, a lapse probably attributable to the same mentality of "fight death at all costs." The result of this omission is that hundreds of doctors call OCME each year and say, as though they had not been through four years of medical school, "Okay, my patient is dead—what do I do now?"

Officially the OCME takes reports on about twenty-four thousand out of the approximately seventy thousand people who die each year in the city. Unofficially, our office handles many more deaths than it reports in the informal conversations we call "consults." The agency doesn't keep accurate statistics on just how many consults are done, but during the time that I ran the communications and identification units, I estimated that our MLIs handled consults on an additional twenty thousand deaths a year. I estimate that almost half the cases called into OCME did not have to be reported because they were natural and expected.

By the end of my first month as a trainee MLI, I knew more about hospital deaths and the reporting of them than did most of the doctors on the other end of the telephone calls. Which was why, when a doctor called to report a death, my first task was always to figure out whether the doctor was calling because the case was reportable or because he or she had no idea what to do. Experienced MLIs develop a sixth sense that enables us to divine why a doctor is calling, and a method of guiding practitioners through the call. I learned to ask questions in a sequence that quickly cut to the chase, such as, "Why did the patient come to the hospital?" It was necessary for me to take control of these conversations because if a clinician were left to ramble, they would tell me in painful detail about every aspect of the patient's health leading up the death. Their inability to get to the point was not entirely their fault because after a patient has been around a hospital for month or so, the clinician who has been treating that patient tends to forget the initial reason for the patient's admission. Moreover because of the regular rotation of the hospital's house staff, the physician who is reporting the death to me may only have treated the decedent for a few days or even a few hours before the death.

Many of these phone calls from confused physicians included the doctor saying such silly things as, "the patient died of cardiopulmonary arrest." After hearing this, I would always say, "Okay, the patient's heart and lungs stopped functioning, but what caused the cardiopulmonary arrest? Was he shot in the head with a bazooka?" Here my deliberately fantastical illustration would generally cause the physicians to laugh and immediately recognize that what I was searching for was an underlying cause for the CPA. The physician would then tell me about the specific *underlying* disease or trauma that caused the death so that together we could make a decision about whether the death was natural or whether it was an ME case.

The sheer volume of such interactions led me to start teaching incoming house staff at the orientations held each year by local hospitals. Unfortunately I was an army of one in the service of this cause, since OCME itself seemed not very interested in this type of "missionary" educational work. Don't get me wrong: no one at the agency prevented me from going out and giving these lectures, but at the same time, no other MLIs joined me in the task, nor were they encouraged to do so from above.

Ultimately, a physician's inability to make a final diagnosis doesn't affect only how many phone calls MLIs must field. Teaching physicians how to make an accurate diagnosis of death and how to properly reflect that diagnosis on a death certificate provides crucial information on many matters that involve public health. This is not simply an issue for medical and death industry professionals—it affects the general public, and quite directly.

Frequently, a newscaster or an interviewee on a television news program (or in print) will say that so many tens of thousands of people died last year in the United States from breast cancer or that lung cancer is now killing more women than breast cancer. Those statistics come from death certificates.

The fact that so many death certificates are not filled out properly has repercussions beyond any individual certificate. It throws a shadow of doubt over such statements as "the number one cause of death in the United States is atherosclerotic heart disease (ASHD)." The reason that ASHD is the "leading cause" is not that we eat too much fast food, though of course we do. Rather, the reason is that doctors put ASHD down on death certificates more often than they put down any other cause of death—and not always because it is the actual cause. In dealing with thousands of doctors over the years, I came to understand that they very quickly learn that ASHD is a good diagnosis to put down on a death certificate because it won't raise red flags with the local ME or coroner's office. Red flags mean the doctors will be bothered with having to resubmit the death certificate with corrections for as many times as it takes them before they get it accepted as correct.

Why bother trying to accurately describe the death as caused by pneumonia, if that diagnosis is guaranteed to generate at least two or three calls to you for more specific information? The person at the ME's office or the coroner's office will ask, "What type of pneumonia, bacterial or viral?" "Left lung or right?" "Was there underlying weakness in the lungs?" To avoid these questions, all across the United States senior medical residents are teaching junior residents a dirty little secret: put down ASHD on the "cause of death" line and those pesky people at the ME's office won't annoy you and the case will go away.

While autopsies would find the exact cause of death, each year in this country, less than *10 percent* of deaths are autopsied, according to the latest annual Vital Statistics summary published by the United States Department of Health and Human Services. That means that 90 percent of the time the cause of death listed on death certificates is either some clinician's best guess, or worse, a diagnosis of convenience. This is a problem for the general public because vital statistics are only vital if they are accurate. The causes of death from each and every death certificate issued in the United States are compiled yearly. The data in the certificates are taken as gospel and are used by the Centers for Disease Control (CDC), the National Institutes of Health (NIH), the federal Department of Health and Human Services, and a host of other organizations as the basis for, among other things, tracking treatments and doling out research dollars. How can those institutions legitimately use this data as the basis of their calculations if for one reason or another the data is tainted?

This is a national disgrace and a dangerous one, but, fortunately, it's not hard to fix. I suggest that we begin at the medical school level, teaching students the importance of vital statistics and how to properly diagnose and report a death.

Not only are these more accurate diagnoses of death better for public health and medical legal jurisprudence, but they're also useful in advancing clinical medicine as well—which is something that we have witnessed in recent years with the epidemic of what is known as SIDS. To help clinicians diagnose and prevent this terrible killer of babies, MLIs in New York fill out a twenty-four-page questionnaire regarding each SIDS death scene—and we do it right in the place where the baby died, with the grieving parents. This is an awful process for the parents and for the MLIs, but we do it and help the parents through it, because of the great potential value of the information being collected. From such interview questionnaires and the information they contain, clinicians have been able to advise parents how to position their infants while they sleep to reduce the risk of SIDS—babies should sleep on their backs. Another such recommendation for parents emerging from the information gathered is that using a pacifier may lower their babies' risk of SIDS by an even larger margin than having them sleep on their backs.

One reason I had been bold enough to try to teach doctors about reporting deaths was that teaching in-house was a large part of my job as a supervising MLI. I trained recruits to OCME—MLIs, MEs, and other professionals. Often, as luck would have it, this training involved some unforgettable death scenes.

While I was training a young female medical student, we were called to a wooded area (one of the few in Manhattan), in the Dyckman area. It was a greensward used for walking dogs and for other, less innocent purposes. A dog walker had come upon an abandoned van, sitting on its axles, with weeds and grass growing up into it. The man's dog had smelled something inside, and had drawn him near to the van. Inside, he had glimpsed a body and had called 911.

My trainee and I went into the van, and indeed found a body in an advanced state of decomposition. It was necessary to take it outside to examine it, so I said to her, "I'll take the legs, you take the arms, and we'll carry it out."

We both pulled, the body started to move—and the head came off, rolling across her foot, and around the floor of the van. The student screamed—a very loud and anguished scream—and ran outside. The cop on duty burst in, revolver drawn, ready to rescue us both from an unseen assailant.

Outside, and trying not to laugh, I attempted to get the trainee to calm down.

She couldn't. She ran to the edge of the area, stamped her feet up and down like a little girl and shouted, "That's the most disgusting thing that's ever happened to me!"

I laughed and laughed, and couldn't stop laughing even in the car on the way back to the office. I did, however, manage to stop laughing long enough to order that the body be brought to OCME for an autopsy. I believed that the decedent had been a derelict who had lived inside the abandoned van and died there of natural causes, rather than having been the victim of foul play, but only an autopsy could confirm this hypothesis.

The next day, I was out in the field when I received a call from one of our MEs, a man with a pronounced British accent. "That body you found at Dyckman yesterday," he began, "Had it a head?" (It wasn't that silly of a question. On other occasions, we've found bodies that had been decapitated to prevent identification.)

"Yes, it had a head," I responded. "Maybe it's in the morgue fridge on the floor." A search of the premises revealed no body-less head floating about. Since the head from the van had evidently not arrived at OCME with the body, I telephoned the county morgue supervisor whose employees transport bodies for OCME and asked him to inquire about the lapse with the driver of that particular run.

The results of his inquiry came back as follows: "Duh, you told us to pick up the body, but you didn't mention the head, so we left it there."

"Go back and finish the job. Pick up the head and bring it in. Please."

The medical student, after this unforgettable initiation, conquered her disgust, and went on to become a pathologist and to work for OCME. She is now one of the top MEs in the Bronx office.

Another doctor who worked his first field case with me is Mark Flomenbaum. Mark came to OCME in the early 1990s, already a board-certified pathologist who had completed his residency, and with it, a four week stint at an ME's office, but he had never been out in the field. Early in his forensic training at OCME, he was assigned to me, and the call we caught first was to a residential hotel on the Upper West Side. It was one step above a flophouse, but it was a small step. A woman had been found dead in a very small room, wedged underneath a wooden cot. As we entered the scene, we were told this was a homicide, but the body had not been discovered for some time and was quite decomposed. The room was so tiny that in order to examine the victim, I had to stand the cot up on its end, against the wall. The space was not large enough to properly accommodate the curious Mark and me, so I asked him to move aside. I examined the body and narrated to him what I was doing and what I was finding. Having confirmed that this was a homicide, which meant that the body would need to be brought in and autopsied, I stood up and prepared to go. Mark moved away from the wall; but he had not been leaning against the wall itself; rather, he had been leaning against the underside of the upended bed, and as he came off it, you could hear his coat peel wetly away. His clothes dripped with, and reeked of, the decomposition fluids. He stunk so badly that we threatened to refuse to have him ride back to OCME in the car with us. We eventually relented, but during the ride back to the office, we tortured him for his odoriferous condition. Despite this rather rude introduction, Mark and I became friends; he finished his training, became an ME for New York, and worked for many years for OCME.

Amy Mundorff, our anthropologist, had similarly been working for OCME for a while, inside the offices, before going out on her first field trip with me. It, too, was rather unusual. In response to a call, we arrived at a brownstone in Greenwich Village to find two uniformed officers, veterans, standing outside and giggling.

"What's so funny?" I asked.

They told me. They had responded to a call about a very bad odor coming from a ground-floor apartment in the back. They had a rookie with them, a very green rookie, and when the apartment could not be entered from the front, they sent him around to the back to go in through a window. The rookie went to the back, broke the window, which was rather high, and stepped inside the apartment. But his first step was onto a glass coffee table, which shattered under his weight. Off balance, his second step landed his foot smack in the abdomen of the deceased man—a very squishy abdomen, since the man had been dead for some time and was a decomposed mess. The rookie's foot went deep into that abdomen. He was so horrified and grossed out that he ran out the front door of the apartment, putrefaction fluids flinging off his foot. He ran past the veterans, down the street and out of sight, and had not been seen since. An hour later, the veterans were still giggling. "He'll come back eventually," they guessed. I wasn't so certain.

Amy and I entered the apartment and looked around. Because of the shattered glass, the bloody footprints, and so on, it looked for all the world as though it could have been the scene of a push-in robbery during which the robber had killed the apartment resident. Had we not known of the rookie's adventures in breaking in—and out—I might have been tempted to guess that this had been a homicide instead of what it was, a natural death, with some pretty significant "postmortem artifact" (a fancy way of saying the cop really messed up the scene).

Amy's only comment on the scene was, "What you do is disgusting. Bones are much cleaner."

That was before she realized that the bones brought into OCME for identification often contained soft tissues along with them—sometimes, very soft.

A while later, I smelled a rather awful odor emanating from Amy's office at OCME and wandered in. A very large pot was boiling on a portable stove, and in it there was a head; she was boiling it to finish denuding it of flesh. I wrinkled my nose and made some comment about how wretched this was.

"Care for some soup?" she needled.

Because I did so well in training people, I became for a time the *de facto* MLI training officer of OCME. It was a good fit. I was the supervising MLI for Manhattan, and all our incoming MLIs would attend courses at headquarters and go out to death scenes in Manhattan, so they were in my bailiwick anyway. I enjoyed training people. Many incoming MLIs and MEs had been clinicians, and I construed their overarching task as learning to think in forensics terms. What's the difference? A clinician thinks about distal events, about end results; a forensician thinks in terms of proximal events, the events that *started* the ball rolling—the first thing that happened. The clinician's natural habitat is the emergency room, the hospital floor, or the like—a place where when a guy goes into cardiac arrest, that's what they treat, watching the vital signs, giving drugs, and performing other interventions. If he gets well, terrific; if he dies, he's no longer their problem. The clinician does not worry about what the person was doing at the time he began to die; the forensics expert does. For an average MLI or ME, completing the arc from thinking in clinical terms to thinking wholly in forensics terms takes about a year.

In 1997, on the retirement of the previous director, I became director of identifications for OCME. Although this was a promotion of sorts, I received no raise in salary, continuing at the rate of a supervising MLI—the only difference was that now, I was a real manager. Previously, I had supervised the MLIs, but that was more of a collegial task; we MLIs treated each other as equals, even though some of us were more experienced than others. As director of identifications, I had to manage the communications unit and five identification units (one for each borough), all of which were staffed by clerks and other bureaucratic personnel. In hierarchical terms, I reported to the director of investigations, putting me on a track that would eventually lead me, I hoped, to achieve that position some day.

I had been director of identifications for four years when the events of September 11, 2001, provided the OCME organization and me with the greatest challenge of my life, identifying the victims of the terrorist attacks.

TEN

BEFORE THE ATTACKS on the World Trade Center, the largest number of simultaneous fatalities the modern OCME had handled came from a mid-air collision over Queens in 1960, in which 134 people died, and from a fire at the Happy Land Social Club in 1990, in which 87 people died. In our disaster planning exercises before 9/11, we had envisioned events of that scale—and confronted a few, including the crash of US Air Flight 405, which slipped off an icy runway at LaGuardia Airport in March 1992, killing 28 passengers and crew members.

On September 11, 2001, it quickly became clear to us, from what we knew of the Trade Center's population during a business day, that the death toll would be far in excess of anything we had ever expected. Although the initial estimates of up to 30,000 fatalities quickly and happily plummeted—what a blessing that the strikes had come before the full complement of workers had arrived at the towers that morning—we were still faced with a task of monumental proportions: processing and identifying the remains of those thousands who did die. Not only was the scale of the disaster unique, but it set for us a series of logistical challenges that would change forever the way OCME conducted its business—the way New York City counted its dead.

Within an hour of the second tower's collapse, I began trying to wrap my head around these challenges.

I realized, almost at once, that we were about to be flooded with what amounted to information from two different sources: the postmortem (data from the remains themselves) and the antemortem (descriptions and details about the victims provided by their family members). As in a death investigation, it would be our job to combine everything we learned from both those sources to enable us to identify each victim. Only now we would be doing so with thousands of victims at once.

The first thing we had to do, I knew, was set up a receiving area—really, a receiving *system*—for bodies and remains. The call went out for refrigerated trucks, and two came almost immediately, one from a vendor at the Fulton Fish Market in Lower Manhattan, something that would have been funny on any other day. These first two trucks (eventually we would use twenty-four of them) were stationed right outside the office's receiving bay on Thirtieth Street, east of First Avenue. Remains arriving from Ground Zero would first go into these trucks. When we were ready for them, they would be taken through processing.

To complete the receiving system, I proceeded into the morgue, still accompanied by Dave Eibert, commanding officer of NYPD's Missing Persons Unit, Mark Flomenbaum, the first deputy chief medical examiner, and Bob Shaler, head of OCME's DNA lab. In addition, our group had swelled to include an entourage of around fifteen interested coworkers. Taking a marker, some paper, and tape, I began to designate areas around the mortuary for the various stations we would need by sticking signs on the walls designating a particular spot for each station, including Fingerprints, Evidence Recovery, DNA collection, X-rays, Dental, Examination/Autopsy, and Anthropology. Some areas didn't have a room or niche of their own, just a wide length of hallway. And so the basic structure of the system was in place. We would receive and first examine the remains outside on the street and then take them into the building for processing.

The OCME is fortunate to have a terrific working relationship with the NYPD, and within half an hour of the disaster, our agency's liaison to the local precinct had made contact and was assured that uniformed officers were on their way. By 10:00 A.M., the NYPD had closed Thirtieth Street to pedestrian and vehicular traffic, so we were able to set up our triage station outside on the street near the refrigerated trucks.

The first step in the identification process was what we thought of as triage. An ME and an anthropologist would examine the contents of each body bag as they came off the trucks—first to make sure that what had been sent to us were remains, and then to determine if the remains were human.

Triage is a process commonly associated with hospitals, as doctors try to separate and prioritize patients before treatment. The situation we faced was similar: the material that arrived in our care after the attacks was so badly damaged and fragmented that firefighters and police officers working in the Ground Zero recovery efforts found it difficult to differentiate remains from other matter—from pulverized concrete, for example, which strongly resembles cremated human remains. "When in doubt, bag it and send it up," we told them—and the result was that our triage table saw all manner of items arrive, some of them downright bizarre.

One such item, rescued from the trash pile, sits on my desk to this day: a set of plastic novelty crooked teeth, yellow and gnarly, clearly from the desk of some office prankster. From time to time, I glance at the choppers and wonder about the person who owned them. Did he or she perish that day? Whoever it was must have had a juvenile sense of humor not unlike my own. I hope he or she survived; perhaps it's you—in which case I hope you'll give me a call.

Once the triage team pronounced an item to be remains, the next step was to determine if they were human. Yes, human: there were a large number of restaurants and food service shops in the WTC complex, and several caterers. We received some "remains" that were soon labeled by our triage people as food items—poultry, pork, chicken, and beef.

Some remains were so small or so badly damaged that triage was unable to verify by examination if they were human or not; in such instances, the remains were treated as human until the DNA lab could make a final determination.

Looking back now from the end of the process, I realize that since not all the remains yielded usable DNA, there might still be a bone or two from a chop or steak mixed in among the unidentified remains. If that is the case, so be it—far better to have kept everything than to have discarded what might yet be identified as human remains, and with them the possibility of an identification that could bring comfort to a grieving family.

The remains confirmed as human were brought from triage to stations within the building, and after processing to an ever-enlarging storage facility. Not all the remains, though, were stored together. Personnel from NYPD and FDNY who were stationed with us at the morgue demanded that any police officer's or firefighter's remains be lodged separately from civilian remains. I had reservations about this practice, on grounds of both practical requirements and social sensibilities; I was reluctant to accept a process that suggested that civilian dead should be treated with any less regard than the uniformed services.

But my attitude slowly changed as I watched the cops and firefighters honor their fallen comrades by treating their remains with an almost religious reverence. There was a long tradition of such reverence in the uniformed services, I learned, dating back at least to the Roman Empire, whose fallen soldiers were brought home on their shields. Even during normal times in New York City, a police officer or firefighter who dies in the line of duty receives an elaborate funeral usually attended by thousands of comrades, sometimes arriving for the occasion from all over the country. Similar traditions exist in most large U.S. cities. As I've come to appreciate, these funerals are a way for surviving service members to say to the world, quite rightly, "What we do is dangerous; what we do is brave; we sacrifice ourselves for the greater good."

Certainly many of the service men and women who responded to the call of duty on September 11 did an extraordinary thing: they ran into the buildings while everyone else who was able was running out. It was this extraordinary, self-sacrificing behavior—which ended up killing so many of the uniformed service men and women—that my

NYPD and FDNY colleagues were honoring by requesting special treatment for their fallen comrades: "Honor these brave men and women because they willingly gave their lives to help others. And honor our profession because we who remain could be similarly called to sacrifice."

However my own feelings on the issue may have changed, many of the civilian families never warmed much to the idea of this special treatment for the uniformed service members. They knew that whenever remains that might belong to a member of service (MOS) were found at Ground Zero, all work at the site came to a halt, a horn was sounded, and an honor guard was formed to salute as the remains were brought out. Then a police escort would escort the remains uptown to OCME where another honor guard would salute as the remains were brought in for processing. Civilian remains received no such treatment. The MOS families were notified immediately after verification of an identification, and sometimes family members were brought in *by helicopter* from outlying areas. Civilian families were notified by the NYPD at a more relaxed pace, and no helicopters were dispatched to bring them in to the city.

Not surprisingly, many civilian families rejected the notion that there were, or should be, two tiers of victims. It was a notion that began on the first day with the separation of the remains, and it created discord between the two groups of families that has continued until today.

Regardless of how the remains were transported or whether they would end up being stored in MOS or civilian trailers, they all went through the same process on arrival. After triage, the remains were assigned a folder with a unique case number and what we called an "escort"—a dedicated person to attend each remain. The idea of an escort was an ad hoc procedure that I came up with that first morning, in an attempt to ensure that no remains would ever end up sitting on a gurney in a hallway without a responsible party available who knew what had been done with them or what yet needed to be done.

At the first station, the Exam/Autopsy table, a gloved and gowned ME carefully went through the remains and described what he or she saw while a scribe, usually a medical student, wrote down the ME's spoken descriptions. Also at the table was a cop from Missing Persons, who took his own notes, and a photographer, who shot both Polaroid and 35mm film. Also present were criminalists from the DNA lab, available to take specimens from the remains and bring them up to the lab.

Together this team recorded all possible postmortem information, starting with the exact time and location where the remains were found, and the hour they arrived at OCME. The postmortem information included a detailed description of the remains, identifying features, type of trauma, and personal property (e.g., jewelry, eyewear, piercings, and any other objects that accompanied the remains).

Our working relationships with many agencies and departments allowed us to have the Fingerprint station manned by NYPD personnel and the Evidence and Property station conducted by the FBI and NYPD. There was also a Dental station where OCME forensic odontologists were in charge. Personnel from various federal agencies roamed the stations, looking for clues to the identities of the attackers and for other evidence about the crime. Some of those agents worked for clandestine intelligence agencies; we learned not to ask them too many questions.

Once we had set up the physical stations down in the morgue, I felt a huge sense of relief. Yet the feeling was fleeting; I was all too aware that processing the remains was only half of the postmortem work ahead of us.

That first morning, before any bodies arrived, I left the morgue and headed back upstairs to the first floor (the administrative level) to start addressing the other half of the work—the paperwork—before the coming informational flood overwhelmed us. No one yet knew how many people had died, or how many remains we might have to identify. The initial rumors of 30,000 deaths were revised downward quickly, but even a month after the event, the predicted number of dead still hovered at 6,000. The eventual death toll, 2,749, was amazingly low, given that up to 50,000 people worked in the towers every day. For all the tragedy involved, it's worth noting that the emergency response to the WTC attacks was also the greatest *rescue* of civilians in modern history—a fact that should bring pride and comfort to the families of the brave men and women who died during the effort.

So, the paperwork was my arena, and as soon as I felt that the morgue process was under control, I began designing an information flow system that would meet the unique challenge of working with such a massive influx of new cases. Each remain would be given its own disaster folder, containing every possible piece of information connected with that remain: intake forms, evidence and property forms, body charts and diagrams, and requisition forms for sending specimens up to our various laboratories. From the outset, we constructed the process in a way that insisted on zero tolerance for anything getting lost or shunted aside. We even included checklists to help ensure that each remain went through the appropriate stages of the identification system. We set up an assembly line for producing the folders, but even when it was working at top speed, WTC remains were arriving at the office so rapidly that they sometimes outpaced our new-folder bucket brigade.

Of course, OCME's regular work did not stop just because of 9/11, and we were also keenly aware of the need to distinguish the WTC remains from the unrelated cases that still arrived, in normal fashion, every day. For that matter, especially in those early days, it was unclear whether the United States might be attacked again soon. So Tom Brondolo, OCME's deputy commissioner for administration, came up with another innovation, a system that assigned a unique "Disaster Manhattan" (DM) case number to each remain, allowing us to differentiate the WTC remains from the other dead. The last thing we wanted was confusion in the morgue; the numbering system helped to prevent that. Tom printed a thousand sheets of color-coded stickers with DM numbers, and as I carried the first batch of stickers to the Identification Office, the numbers of dead represented by these sheets of labels made me feel sick all over again at the magnitude of the disaster.

The next stage was to transfer the information we had gathered into a computerized system. All the precious information we were collecting by hand, and recording on paper, would be useless if it just lay in folders—

especially when it came to the daunting task of collating dispersed remains and looking for possible clues that could lead to a positive identification. My mind raced with possibilities: I imagined a hand being found amid the rubble and that there would be a ring on that hand, a plain yellow band bearing the inscription "JD & JD forever." I further imagined Jane Doe coming in, reporting her husband John Doe missing in the Trade Center disaster, and filling out a missing persons report mentioning that he wore such a ring on the fourth finger of his left hand. Needless to say, the chances of solving that puzzle would be far greater if our team were able to search a computerized database of such clues—a convenience that was far less necessary under normal circumstances, but which became crucial with the volume of unsolved cases we suddenly faced after 9/11.

But there was one hitch: as far as I knew, no one in the forensic field had developed such a database—certainly not at OCME. So Tom started the process from scratch, using a program called Dataease that was especially good for rapid development of "user interfaces"—the screens used to enter and view data. We set up four data-entry stations in our conference room; we knew we'd need more before long, but we had to start somewhere. I commandeered a hodgepodge crew of identification staff, MLIs, and even a forensic dentist to staff the stations; by the time the first folder came up from the morgue later that day, we were ready.

As I ran around the building, fueled with adrenaline, I must have looked like a dervish to some of my coworkers, as I tried to be everywhere at once. I issued peremptory orders to staffers and volunteers who had begun to flood in: *You go to this station. You enter that data. Here's how you enter the information.* Yet everyone was so willing to help that my commands met with few objections.

And the help came from outside, too: We received unsolicited calls offering gloves, gurneys, office supplies, refrigerated trucks, food—anything they could imagine us needing—in addition to volunteers. I asked someone at the communications unit to keep a log of each one of the thousands of offers of help we received. You had to be careful what you asked for: One day, in an OCME hallway, I muttered to myself, "We need some decent copiers around here." Someone overheard me, and presto, within a day or so, two $30,000 copiers appeared in our offices. I never found out who provided them, and I don't think we ever received a bill.

At one point during that day, I heard someone mention that OCME actually had an official Mass Disaster Plan, devised to help the office cope with high-fatality incidents—that is, events in which ten or more people were killed.

I never even opened that document; it would have been useless in a tragedy of this scale. *How quickly we despise today,* I thought, *the amateurs we were yesterday.*

As it happened, the first body to arrive was someone I knew of from news reports and by reputation. Case number DM-01-0001 was Father Mychal Judge, a Franciscan friar who was a chaplain to the FDNY. But only Father Judge and a few more of the first bodies through our doors were relatively intact. We very rapidly noted a horrifying change in the condition of the remains. Even seasoned MEs who had years of experience became dismayed as body bag after body bag of pulverized human remains came through. We saw every conceivable and quite a few impossible-to-imagine types of trauma: remains that ranged in size from whole bodies, to small pieces the size of a dime, in conditions that ranged from burned to blasted, shredded to crushed. That first day, some of the remains actually arrived still smoking and warm from the fires.

I stationed myself in the intake area and personally logged in the first thirty-two remains longhand in a large bound record book. I handled these myself because I wanted to be sure the system was working properly, from the holding trucks to the triage to the various stations and on to the storage trucks. This processing system that we threw together in an hour worked well that day and would continue to function well until May 2002, when the last of the WTC remains were processed.

After the first few days, we knew that the OCME effort would focus exclusively on identification. Other than the identity of the victims, there was not much mystery about the cause of death in this homicide investigation. Everyone in the world who owned a television had witnessed the crime, and within seventy-two hours, we also knew who had done it. All that was left was to determine who had perished. This one-dimensional aspect of the investigation thrust OCME into the forefront of public consciousness as never before in the agency's history. So we turned all of our efforts toward a seemingly impossible goal: identifying every victim we possibly could, no matter how difficult it might be or how much time it might take. The public needed us to do this, Dr. Hirsch was determined to do it, and as director of identifications, I was committed to devoting all our energies and resources to the identifications.

To get a sense of the magnitude and difficulty of the identification task, consider this statistic: we would eventually recover almost twenty thousand body parts and fragments from Ground Zero and the surrounding area. Most of them were in terrible condition, having been exposed to very high heat, to water, and to other pressures that rendered almost useless our traditional identification methods. Under the prolonged exposure to high heat, even the DNA in the recovered bones began to deteriorate; in many instances, it was too far gone for us to analyze.

The city set up two operations to recover remains, one at the site of the disaster, the second at a recently closed landfill on Staten Island with the unfortunate name Fresh Kills. I was not at the meetings that led to Mayor Rudolph Giuliani's decision to have the rubble from Ground Zero loaded onto trucks, then onto barges, taken across the bay, and finally spread out and sifted through on a garbage dump. It was part of the city's grand and noble effort to retrieve every possible bit of human remains, but for a number of reasons, the location could not have been more ill-chosen. The name of the site alone should have made any responsible public official shudder. Still, the rubble—more than a million tons in all—did have to be examined, and there were further remains being found in it.

With identifications piling up, that first week went by in a blur of frenetic activity. For the first three days after the disaster, I worked in the same clothes, without going home, and with only a nap now and then. Part of my job was to organize many of those who volunteered to assist us—among them the people from the Disaster Mortuary Operational Response Team (DMORT), who soon began arriving to help. DMORT is a national volunteer organization of MLIs, funeral directors, and morticians who mobilize to help local officials during disasters as part of FEMA's disaster-relief resources. In addition, every consultant we'd ever had at OCME came to help, as did coroner's and ME's office personnel from around the country. We needed them all. One fellow drove from New Mexico, and slept in his car for four days before he was able to get in to see me. He ended up working for us for several months, for no pay, sleeping on a cot we arranged for him next door at NYU. I learned much later that folks from his small hometown had taken up a collection to help him stay in New York as long as he did.

The postmortem information we culled from the remains was not enough by itself to make positive identifications. We also needed *ante-mortem* information (data about the missing people), which began streaming in from the families within hours and soon grew into a separate database of astonishing size. Here's why: anyone who was in Manhattan in those weeks after 9/11 saw the missing-persons photos and pleas plastered to any available surface—walls, lampposts, or bus stop shelters. That same set of information reached us, and more: we were flooded with photos, ID cards, X-rays, dental records, toothbrushes, hairbrushes, teddy bears, and other items that families thought would help us identify their loved ones. Every single item had to be accepted, cataloged, and cross-referenced, so the information would be useful. At the Family Assistance Center, thousands of family members, significant others, coworkers, neighbors, and sometimes just plain busybodies filled out seven-page Victim Identification Profiles forms in longhand, providing us with every speck of information that might be helpful, from descriptions of rings or other jewelry to tattoos and even the type of shoes a victim usually wore. "This was the shirt he wore at the barbecue this weekend," they would say. "It was still in the laundry.

Can you get DNA from this?" Or, "Here is her dentist's name and number. She just went last week because she wanted to have her teeth whitened for her wedding next month. They should have her dental records."

And then there were the photographs—those powerful, heartbreaking photos, usually of groups or family gatherings, with the "missing" person circled. "Have you seen anyone who looks like him?" a family member would ask; but their eyes would say, "Please, don't *you* find him; let him be in a hospital somewhere, alive." How do you tell a grieving, frightened widow, "No, we haven't seen him. I have seen only pieces of what used to be people"?

Early in October 2001, three weeks after that terrible September 11, a discovery made far beneath the rubble pile at Ground Zero summoned me from the Incident Command Center at OCME into the field on a collection mission.

High-ranking police officials had shown up at OCME early that Sunday morning to ask if I would come down to the site. A body had been located, four stories under the debris at Ground Zero, where the North Tower had once stood. "We think we found a brother officer," Deputy Inspector Kenny McKeel told me, "but we don't think we can get him out anytime soon. Can you come down and take a look? Maybe you can start the ID process." Kenny's description of the situation, in combination with my understanding of how quickly decomposition takes its toll on bodies, galvanized me. I informed the staff of the Incident Command Center that I would be down at Ground Zero for a few hours and jumped in the police car.

I had not been out of the office much during the previous weeks and the ride downtown revealed that the city still had an urgent, chaotic feel to it, which even a first-time visitor would have recognized as a city in a state of emergency: traffic lanes reserved for emergency and other official vehicles, and every street along the route to Ground Zero lined with people. Hundreds and hundreds of them held up signs that said "Thank You" or "God Bless You," and the ones who were not holding signs just applauded and called to us as the car went by. Unable to directly help, they were pouring out their appreciation for the people intimately involved in the recovery effort. They brought tears to my eyes. Their presence, and their good wishes, reinforced the feeling of unity in New York—in the whole country—that would last for many months. Looking back now, almost five years later, I only wish we had held on to a little of that feeling a bit more permanently.

I had been to Ground Zero two weeks earlier, but this time, on arriving there, I was staggered by the scope of the recovery effort, now going at full throttle, working on what the workers called the "Pile." I use the phrase *recovery* effort, since in October of 2001, that was the official label. It had not been easy for the city to stop using the phrase *rescue* effort. As for me, from the moment that the Towers fell, I realized there would be few if any survivors and not many additional rescues. A first public note of realism was sounded on September 18 by Mayor Rudolph Giuliani: "We don't have a substantial amount of hope to offer to people that there is anyone alive there," he told a press conference. "We have to prepare for the overwhelming possibility that finding anyone alive is very, very small." Just then the city was not yet ready to give up hope that by some miracle survivors might be found; but on September 29, the city officially stopped using the term "rescue" and reluctantly switched to "recovery."

Heavier equipment was now being used to shift around the rubble, but otherwise, the change in objective from rescue to recovery was meaningless to the firefighters, police officers, steel workers, and others who toiled ceaselessly around the clock, digging into the Pile. They continued to act as rescue workers.

It is hard for anyone who wasn't at Ground Zero in those chaotic days to fathom the bravery of the people who were physically working on the Pile, spearheading the recovery effort. As I watched, they attacked the rubble with picks, shovels, crowbars, and even with their hands. The big machinery was used mainly for pieces of steel that were far too massive to be moved by human strength. But the smaller debris was removed manually, by workers in long bucket brigades carrying out the material. And they were doing so on a gigantic pile of twisted steel, smashed concrete, and who knew what else, that was *ablaze!* Fires were raging in and under the rubble that reached temperatures in excess of 1,800 degrees Fahrenheit. Many if not most of the police officers and fire fighters digging at the mounds of debris had lost coworkers and close friends. A few like Lee Ielpi, whom I met that day, were even looking for their family members. Lee, a veteran firefighter, was searching for his son, also a firefighter, who was buried somewhere under the rubble. Lee had sworn to his wife that he would not rest until he brought his son home.

Augmenting those brave guys at work on the Pile every day, in conditions of utmost physical and emotional peril, was another group of men for whom the word "brave" is an inadequate adjective. Their task was, if anything, even more dangerous: to go down *into* the Pile on as many as five search and recovery missions daily. Until September 29, they had searched for survivors, and since then had been searching for remains. Their dedication was incredible. They were risking their lives in the effort to recover the *body parts* of a fallen comrade or civilian victim. Those trekking regularly into the inferno were members of New York's Finest (NYPD) and Bravest (FDNY), together with police officers from the Port Authority of New York and New Jersey. In small groups, they went inside, every day for months, looking for human remains.

That Sunday morning, Kenny McKeel brought me over to one such group, led by Joe Blozis, a sergeant from NYPD's CSU, whom I knew well from years of working cases together. "Not to worry, you're in good hands," Kenny said, and I knew that was true. Joe is a giant of a man, around six feet four inches and broad as a barn door. He took me to a supply area where we suited up. Tough overalls, boots, goggles, a hard hat with a lantern, heavy duty work gloves and, to complete the outfit, a double-barreled full-face respirator that the guys said was guaranteed to keep out most of the contaminants known to be floating around the site.

Thus equipped, our group of six men, including me, was ferried to the edge of the site in a roofless vehicle called a Gator, which looked like a giant golf cart borne by six overstuffed, knobby tires. Joe was grinning behind his mask. "You all right, doc?" As an employee of the ME's office you constantly get called doc, whether or not you're an MD. You get tired of explaining that you're not and simply perk up when some-body says, "Hey, doc."

"Yeah," I responded, "let's just get this over with." Actually, of course, I was terrified, but somehow managed to move my feet, and we started walking the hundred yards or so across the top of the rubble pile to where we would begin our descent.

A hundred yards is not too great a distance when you're strolling along Fifth Avenue, but it's endless when you're crossing the equivalent of a debris field in an urban war zone. Every step was fraught with dan-ger because none was on a flat surface. I stepped from beam to beam, from one large chunk of concrete to another. Razor-sharp pieces of steel poked out at me from every direction, often hardly visible in the gray smoke pouring up from the ground. Along the way, we passed a large, golden-colored metal ball that I recognized with a start as a sculpture that had graced the plaza between the two towers. It was the only recognizable artifact on the Pile.

After reaching the center of the debris field, one by one we crawled backward through a small hole, tied together like spelunkers, to begin our descent. Our way was lit by the lanterns we carried and by the bare bulbs that had been strung on endless extension cords. Under the Pile were a surprising number of cavernous pockets, and once inside one, I could sometimes see forty or fifty feet around me. My experienced guides seemed at home, moving confidently about as though they knew where they were going; I, however, felt like I was moving slowly in a nightmare of frightening, surreal jumbles of twisted wreckage, between house-sized agglomerations of metal, stone, and concrete, each indis-tinguishable from the next. After we had descended about twenty feet through these labyrinths, I felt like an ant crawling around a junkyard.

Only this was no junkyard, it was a graveyard, a giant tomb. In the dim light, I could make out spray-painted numerals, arrows, and other symbols, the fruits of previous expeditions. Some of the markings, I soon realized, staked out areas where remains had been found. Other marks showed egress and exit points. Some I simply could not deci-pher, but I didn't ask my fellow spelunkers about them as conversation among us was virtually impossible at first, partly because of the masks we wore but also because of the thunderous noise above our heads. It came from mobile cranes rumbling around the site, tearing at the rubble, sending pieces of it flying about and crashing down. When one of those huge cranes stirred, or moved a particularly large piece of rubble, dust would drift down on us and the wreckage we were walking through would creak and shift eerily, as though it was some special effect in an Indiana Jones movie.

But it wasn't Hollywood, it was real, and I was engaged in a job that terrified me. Today I'm somewhat amazed that I was able to do it, but the can-do, we-Americans-are-helping-one-another spirit of the moment assisted me to get through my fears, as it assisted so many others.

We descended farther, nearing the victim. The noise began to subside. After squeezing through yet another narrow concrete-and-steel passageway, we popped out into the largest open space I had yet seen, and the sight left me awestruck. After a few seconds, I realized that we were in what had once been an underground parking garage for the Port Authority police. The north side of it was virtually intact and two Port Authority police cars sat there in their assigned parking spots, untouched by the devastation around them except for being covered by five inches of the ubiquitous gray powder; but for the dust, it could have been a car showroom. Here we were able to stand upright. We walked normally to the end of the room, turned the corner, and entered a staircase—at which point any semblance of normalcy again disappeared. An enormous steel H-beam had pierced the ceiling of the stairwell on its plunge downward, and its momentum had been arrested only a few inches before it touched the steps. It had become a giant metal stalactite, a mute testament to the unimaginable forces unleashed on that terrible day. We squeezed around it, one by one, walked up six steps to the first landing and turned as though to go up the next flight—but there were no more stairs. The Pile had flattened them, and protruding from the mess of that non-stairway was a booted left foot. From the looks of the boot, it belonged to a uniform, possibly that of a Port Authority officer who had gone down into the parking lot in the minutes after the attacks trying to evacuate anyone still left inside, only to be caught on the stairs by the collapsing building.

It had taken half an hour and the efforts of five other people to get me here. Now it was time for me to do my job. With help from my comrades-in-arms, I cut open his boot and severed his pinkie toe, which I dropped into a DNA specimen container. I took the entire toe, bone and all, because I was worried that his soft tissues had already decomposed too far to provide useable DNA. I paused for a moment before we left, feeling deeply moved and choked up as I imagined this brave man's last few moments. I hoped that we would be able to identify him, and that his family would find some peace in the knowledge that he had been doing his job to the end.

Eventually, the victim was identified. He was, indeed, a Port Authority police officer, and the rest of his remains were brought out and given to the family for burial.

ELEVEN

ON THE STREET surrounding our office building, a tent city had sprung up, covering both sides of Thirtieth Street from First Avenue to the FDR Drive at the river's edge, housing an incredible assortment of city, state, and federal agencies, as well as a chapel and a large mess tent where the Salvation Army served up as many as 1,200 meals a day. Hundreds of remains were being processed at a time, a pace we had been maintaining since the disaster occurred. The body-receiving system that we had set up that first day was functioning smoothly and no longer in need of constant tinkering. It was operating twenty-four hours a day.

Inside our building, in the main-floor-level conference room, our Incident Command Center was also transformed. Thirty-five feet by fifteen feet, it was now packed with dozens of people and with thirty computer terminals. The database system had to be up and running on a continuous basis; yet we also constantly needed to make adjustments to its software programs to accommodate all the information we were receiving and to make use of the data once it had been entered. Normally, computer systems are shut down so that programmers can open the software, make changes, and test them out; only after that do they return the system to full functioning. Fixing a "live" system, on the fly, constituted what our outside consultants called "extreme programming."

Prior to 9/11, the entire OCME Information Management Department consisted of two people. To support OCME's response to the

WTC attacks, the office quickly turned to outside contractors and used many different computer experts in various areas. Four of these vendors worked directly with me in the Incident Command Center and became integral members of our team. The first keyboard jockey to arrive was Adrian Jones, a British software developer—and Dataease expert, it turned out—who happened to be attending a convention in the United States at the time of the attacks. Tom Brondolo, OCME's deputy commissioner for administration, knew that Adrian was at that convention and got word to him that we really needed his help.

Within a few days of the attack, I returned from a trip to the Family Assistance Center to find a tall, slender fellow with a mop of dark, curly hair sitting at one of the computers, typing blindingly fast on the keyboard in a rhythmic pattern, as though playing a piano. He finished with a dramatic flourish and turned, realizing I was standing over him. "Hallo," he said in a clipped British accent. "I'm Jones, Adrian Jones, at your service."

"Pleased to meet you, Mr. Bond—I mean, Mr. Jones." No, I didn't say that; I only wish I had. But this introduction proved to be the start of a wonderful partnership: I knew what business the office needed to conduct, and Adrian knew his computers. Together we spent countless hours building a data management system nimble enough to absorb every twist and turn the disaster and its aftermath threw at us. Having planned to be in the States for only the few days of the conference, Adrian had with him just a small overnight bag. When we asked him to stay on and help us, he agreed. But he would need to buy a few more pieces of clothing since he stayed on for two years, becoming a critical part of the OCME effort. Shortly after Adrian arrived, we were joined by two more Dataease experts, Al Munoz and Don Metzger, and then by Naeem Ullah, a colleague of Adrian's from the same London-based company.

Over at Pier 92, the Emergency Operations Center was chock-full of teams that flew in from Microsoft and other large information-technology companies. Tom Brondolo invited the consulting teams over to OCME to see if they could help with our operation. Unfortunately, almost all of them had to be sent packing: many of them wanted to do three studies and a planning document for every little task they *might* be assigned. They meant well, but if they'd been our main team, we'd still be holding meetings.

In contrast, our four gunslingers, as they liked to call themselves, attacked the problems directly and with amazing speed. They got the job done.

The Incident Command Center also evolved in terms of function as we added more tasks to those we were already doing. New ones included arranging shipping and travel for remains and DNA samples, assisting families in various ways, and maintaining a twenty-four-hour-a-day telephone hotline. As the manager of the Incident Command Center, I had to categorize in my mind all the 9/11-related operations we were simultaneously handling, in order to keep them all going at once.

The tasks broke down into five major groups.

The first, of course, was the gathering of postmortem information from the remains, from bloody clothing that came in, and from other personal effects, and processing these through the system. Where and when was the item or part found? At the site or at the landfill? By whom, if that were known? (If it had been found at the site, the grid location was also recorded: FDNY had overlaid a grid map on the entire site, dividing the work areas into seventy-by-seventy-foot squares.) A toe-tag number was assigned at the site, and to this, at the OCME processing area, the remains would then have a DM number added, a DNA number, and a number from Evidence would also be given to any personal property taken from the remains. Sometimes when a body bag was opened at the processing area, three separate parts would be found inside. Each would receive a separate DM number, even though they all had the same toe-tag number. For complex headaches like these, our highly flexible computer program and its ingenious operators proved essential.

The second task was processing the antemortem stream of information that came mainly from the families in the Victim Identification Profiles. At the Family Assistance Center, thousands of these seven-page Victim Identification Profile forms were filled out—on paper—

during interviews with police officials. In addition, important information also came to us from the employers of the victims, from nongovernmental organizations such as the Red Cross and Salvation Army, from foreign governments whose citizens had been killed, and from police departments and AGs' offices across the United States. To transcribe the data, 180 DMORT volunteers sat in an area of the Emergency Operations Center called the blue dot area (because you needed a blue dot on your ID badge to get in) and, working sixty at a time at as many computer stations, entered the information from the Victim Identification Profile forms. Even though we worked around the clock, the task still took almost two months to complete.

Once the information was entered, we faced another Herculean task: "washing" the data, cleaning out errors, and consolidating multiple reports on the same person. In one instance, a man who feared that his brother had been killed in the WTC made eleven such reports. The day after the bombings, he left his home in Baltimore, Maryland, determined to reach New York and either find his brother or report him missing. Aware of how long it might take him to get into New York because of the travel restrictions in the immediate aftermath of the attacks, he started the ball rolling by reporting his brother missing to the Baltimore police. During his journey to New York, this well-meaning man stopped and re-reported his brother as a missing person at least twice more, in different police jurisdictions, and also told the Red Cross and the Salvation Army. On reaching New York City, he made at least a half dozen more reports, for instance at the local police precinct in the area of his brother's residence and then at the Family Assistance Center. When finished, he had created eleven reports about his brother, each with enough variation in detail and spelling to get entered into the database as a unique record with its own case number.

To tease out and eliminate the redundant reports and consolidate the eleven records into one was an enormously time-consuming task. At one point, there were over sixty thousand official missing person reports in our system—which averages out to around twenty-two reports per victim, each of them generated by a well-meaning "reporter" (as we called them) determined to ensure that his friend or family member did not get overlooked.

One aspect of the antemortem stream over which we at OCME had no control was the taking of DNA samples from victims' families. By executive decree from the mayor's office, this was being done by the NYPD. They had argued to City Hall that they knew how to do it and had more manpower available for the task than we did. We at OCME thought this was a bad idea, arguing that collecting DNA samples from families without a medically-trained person present was fraught with potential dangers. We pointed out that we were expert in taking DNA samples, having had loads of experience producing "exemplars" for court cases. Despite our protests, the NYPD managed to keep OCME personnel away from the DNA collection process. In one incident, I later heard, one of our DNA experts tried to sit in on some DNA-collecting sessions with victim families at the Family Assistance Center and was actually escorted out the door by cops.

Our third task, devolving from the first two, was developing a missing persons list. Mass disasters are of two types: Some are classified as "closed universes"; others as "open universes." An example of a closed-universe disaster is a plane crash, where the passenger manifest tells us precisely how many people were on the plane, who they were, and even where they were sitting. An open-universe disaster is one where we do not know how many people were killed nor who they were. The WTC attacks created the mother of all open-universe disasters.

The WTC buildings were not only incredibly large but also completely open to the public, a major tourist destination, and the center of a mass transit hub. The WTC was like a small city, complete with shops, restaurants, and other businesses catering to the public. Messengers, fast-food and flower delivery people, UPS, FedEx, photocopy repairmen—the list was endless. Little wonder that early estimates of the number of dead were so high. There was no way of predicting what the foot traffic in that building actually was.

In developing a missing persons list, the OCME was trying to close the most open of open-universe disasters, in part through the work of a committee whose birth was never mandated by the mayor or by any other ranking city official. It came into being as its members, all charged with the day-to-day tasks of working with the victims or their families, recognized the need for a coordinated effort. The working group that we formed continued to operate for close to three years. Members included Inspector (now Chief) Jerry Quinlan of the NYPD, Deputy Commissioner Tommy Curitore of the Mayor's Community Assistance Unit, Deputy Commissioner Bradford Billet of the Mayor's Commission to the United Nations, and myself. The Fire Department also sent a representative to many of our meetings, and later on police officials working on WTC fraud cases joined our group.

The prime goal of the "Reported Missing" committee was to establish an official list broken down into two major victim categories: Reported Missing and Confirmed Dead. Victims achieved the status of Reported Missing after the committee verified that the missing person report was genuine, that such a person existed and had likely perished. Victims were confirmed dead by one of two mechanisms: (1) after having their bodies identified, (2) in the absence of remains having a death certificate issued by judicial decree. The Confirmed Dead portion of the list became the focus of intense media scrutiny—and we were very careful in adding names to this category because those names inevitably appeared the next morning on the front pages of newspapers around the world.

The plethora of agencies involved and the multitude of pathways onto the list had created a system with too many numbers. A family member would call the police and report a loved one missing; at the end of the conversation, he or she would get a T number that stood for the telephone report. Later the same family would have an interview at the Family Assistance Center and receive a P number for that personal interview. Then OCME would give them a DX number on the judicial decree death certificate, which the family could add to the L number that the Law Department gave them for their affidavit. And so on, and on, and on. A family might easily rack up close to twenty different case numbers reporting one victim; families with multiple victims could have even more.

We knew that if we were ever to get control of the situation and bring together all the different agencies' databases, we'd need a super number to "roll-up" all those other numbers and their associated data into one master database. Part of designing the missing persons list also meant that the committee had to create that super number—called the Reported Missing (RM) number—which encompassed every other number assigned to anything else.

One open secret of the WTC identification effort was that we never accomplished the goal of closing the universe of known victims—that is to say, not everyone who was dead was listed on the missing persons list. We never made any effort to hide this fact, but it received little publicity. I am not speaking of being unable to *identify* everyone. We did not expect to ever do that. Rather, we list compilers knew there were more victims out there than we were able to confirm as missing. In our opinion, this was one of the biggest stories of the WTC, but no one really picked up on it. Those that remained off the missing persons list included victims who had been reported, at least unofficially, but whose names, for one reason or another, we simply could not confirm.

Such was the case when we received reports from grassroots immigration organizations that undocumented workers, primarily in the food service areas of the Trade Center, had perished, but that their names were not being furnished to us because their relatives were afraid of being deported. Part of the problem, which we discovered during our negotiations with community-based groups here in New York, was that terrified family members also living here illegally would not believe that they could safely report their loved one dead without facing deportation. The group of reports that seemed most credible concerned a dozen or so undocumented Mexican food service workers. Together with Brad Billet and his outfit, the mayor's commission to the United Nations, we at OCME tried diligently to reach out to the families of these ghost victims. We even solicited the help of the countries from which the illegal aliens had likely come to the United States so that we could at least list the names of these people who were missing and

181

could be presumed to be among the WTC dead; but these efforts did not bring us many names or much information by which we might have been able to identify particular decedents.

As a result, I believe that there are quite a few casualties of 9/11 whose names are not being recited at the annual memorial services.

The difficulty of identifying the dead forced us into accomplishing a very important task: bringing into being a system for issuing what are called "nonphysical remains" death certificates.

A family or survivor of a decedent must have a death certificate in order to satisfy the requirements of insurance companies, mortgage holders, banks, and a whole host of other entities that control portions of the decedent's property or access to it. Without a death certificate, for example, you can't collect on your loved one's insurance or have access to his or her bank accounts; your mortgage company will likely not be willing to give you a few months grace in which to replace the former breadwinner's income stream and pay the monthly installments—and so on. A certificate would also become the key to unlocking access to the funds set up to aid WTC victims' families.

In normal times, most certificates are issued for deaths in which there are physical remains, that is, for a body. Prior to the WTC tragedy, obtaining a death certificate in New York City without having confirmation of death by means of examining the physical remains was a long and very involved process, one that could often take as much as seven years. You reported the person missing, you exhausted all remedies to locate him or her, you made application to the Surrogate Court—usually with the assistance of a lawyer—and years after the disappearance of your loved one, the Court would direct the OCME and the city's Health Department to issue a "certificate by judicial decree," also known as a "nonphysical remains" death certificate. In the interim, you might well have lost your home, never collected on the insurance from the decedent, and generally entered a long and unpleasant holding pattern.

We at OCME recognized soon after the WTC disaster that the intensity of the collapse and the fires would make it impossible to collect and identify the remains of every victim. We therefore needed to set up a process that would make it possible for the families to receive a death certificate without having the physical remains present, since in many cases the death certificate was the key that would allow them to move on with their lives. This difficult endeavor quickly became our fourth major task.

Four city bureaucracies, the Surrogate Court, the OCME, New York City's Office of Corporation Counsel (its legal department, also known as the Law Department), and the Department of Health (DOH) cooperated wonderfully in setting up a system for obtaining "nonphysical remains" death certificates. Together, we agreed that two affidavits would be created for each decedent. One was to be filled out by the decedent's family, usually under the guidance of an attorney from the Law Department. The New York Bar Association also provided family members free legal assistance in helping them to fill out the affidavits. The "family" affidavit provided us with such information as a wife's recollection that, for example, the husband worked as a trader at the brokerage firm Cantor Fitzgerald, and had gone to work at the WTC that day, as he had done every working day at 8:00 A.M., and had called her from the office twice—once to confirm dinner arrangements, and the second time to tell her that the plane had hit, that he was going to die, and that he loved her and the kids. These affidavits, which arrived at a rate of twenty to sixty a day, contained many such stories that were utterly heartbreaking to read, and the records of such phone calls were simply devastating. It was an incredibly difficult experience, but one that left me amazed by the grace and lovingness demonstrated by the victims before their deaths and the strength that their loved ones displayed in the aftermath.

The second affidavit, which we called the "employer" affidavit, would contain information and evidence supplied by the decedent's company or place of business, including pay stubs and the like. At OCME's and DOH's insistence, the body of these two affidavits had to include the following information: age, race, sex, last known address, years of schooling, military service dates, date of birth, date of death, father's name, mother's maiden name. In some instances, of course, these facts were not immediately available to the families and the searching took precious time. Nonetheless, we insisted on including this information because the nonphysical remains death certificates were going to be no different than the regular "remains" certificate and required these fields be filled out, as well as many other data fields containing all of the pertinent social, demographic, and statistical data that was legally required. The medical portion, the cause of death, "blunt trauma—no physical remains" and manner of death, "homicide," were the same for every certificate. These nonphysical remains certificates were label DX—the D for disaster and the X for "by judicial decree."

One additional line told the entire story of each person in summary—the "How Injury Occurred" section of the certificate. "Firefighter killed while responding to WTC attacks," it would read, or "Passenger aboard American Airlines Flight 11, which was crashed into WTC." Many simply read, "Office worker killed in WTC attacks." A companion box listed whether the victim had been at work at the time of death. This simple fact also could have significant consequences in terms of the type of compensation that a victim's family might receive.

The affidavits were compiled in triplicate, a copy for the Surrogate Court, another for OCME, and a third for the Law Department. After receiving the affidavits, the Law Department dispatched copies simultaneously to the Surrogate Court and the OCME, enabling us to prepare our response while the Court was going through its certification process. This way we would be ready to move once the Court sent over to us a judicial decree that permitted the issuance of a nonphysical remains death certificate. While the Court's own process could take anywhere from a few days to a month, we would take much less time to complete our end. I pledged to Dr. Hirsch that within twenty-four hours of our receipt of a judicial decree we would have a death certificate for the family. It was an ambitious goal, but one that we were able to achieve.

One of the main reasons I was able to keep this promise was a wonderful woman named Katie Sullivan. A sociologist and computer science professor in Oregon, she had joined DMORT a few months before 9/11, even though she had no forensic experience—she simply wanted to help with the computer end of the organization. When the attacks occurred, she was at home watching the events on television like everyone else in America, when suddenly it occurred to her, "Oh, no—I just joined DMORT!"

Before the end of September, she was in New York, deployed by DMORT for what was supposed to be a two-week stint. Initially she was assigned to work upstairs in the DNA lab and did for the first few days, but one day she ended up in my area and her role was transformed in the course of a single meeting—all because she raised her hand.

During a week of all-nighters, Adrian Jones and I had come up with a series of computer screens that would allow us to enter affidavit data and use it to generate a death certificate. The software worked, but when we tried to teach a large group of volunteers and clerical temps how to use it, things quickly went awry. After a few moments of confusion, a hand went up in the back of the room, and a pleasant-faced, supremely calm lady, looking for all the world like the Pacific Northwest "granola girl" that she was, stood up and said, "I teach computers for a living; I get what you're trying to do here. Can I take over?"

Adrian nodded, and I said, "Yup. It's all yours." I stuck around for a few minutes to watch her, became completely impressed, and then got out of her way. By the next day, she was telling me how many workers she needed on each shift. By the third day, she was recommending which workers to retain and which could not do the task. On the fourth day, I placed her in charge of the entire affidavit-entry process. Katie's unique combination of computer skills, sociological training, and willingness to work made her invaluable. She was the quickest study I'd ever met in my life, and when DMORT finally refused to "re-up" her, OCME hired her to be my assistant director. Her husband and cat came to join her in New York, and she kept working.

That appointment allowed me to deal with another developing problem having to do with the DX certificates. Some victim families initially did not want nonphysical remains certificates because they thought that accepting one would mean that we would stop searching for their loved one's remains or stop trying to identify remains as belonging to their loved one.

I talked with many such families, trying to reassure them that we would not stop searching, and that if we did eventually make an identification, we would hasten to replace the nonphysical remains certificate with a physical remains certificate. I stressed that insurance companies and other property guardians would just as readily accept one kind of certificate as the other. Can you imagine any mortgage company in America at that moment in time, refusing to accept a New York City nonphysical remains death certificate, or not granting a WTC-victim family a few months grace on a mortgage payment?

My friend Dr. Steve Schwartz, registrar of the city of New York and head of vital statistics (the division of the Department of Health that issues death certificates), set up an auxiliary shop at our office precisely for the purpose of hurrying along the issuance of the judicial-decree death certificates. We all knew the importance of this matter. Still, some problems remained in the system, stemming from the Surrogate Court's refusal to identify the decedent on the court order beyond using his or her name. For example, we had four decedents named Michael Francis Lynch, two of them firefighters. I tried everything I could to have the Court use our ID numbers—or any other recognizable ID numbers, such as a Social Security tag—to more precisely identify the person for whom the decree was being issued, but it was to no avail. We had to scramble every time a court order came in on a duplicate name.

Eventually, we issued 2,347 nonphysical remains certificates to families of the victims, most of them during a frantic, three-month marathon. Overall, there were 2,749 victims of the mass murder at the WTC, which means that 85 percent of the victim families benefited by receiving a judicial decree certificate. By the time the identification shop shut down, we had identified more than 1,600 (roughly 60 percent) of the victims. In other words, many of the victim families received *both* kinds of certificates, but a large proportion of the identifications happened years after the DX certificates had been issued.

I exclude from these numbers four bodies that we identified and listed as suicides: those remains belonged to the terrorists. This fact is not well-known to the public: four out of the twelve or thirteen terrorists aboard the two planes were actually identified through our process. The positive identifications of the four were made by matching postmortem DNA obtained from body parts found at the site with DNA samples provided to OCME by the FBI. Federal investigators had taken swabbings from places the terrorists were known to have been, such as motel rooms and airport gates. As soon as these remains were identified, the terrorists' remains were segregated from other remains and turned over to Dr. Hirsch. I don't know precisely what was done with those remains, but Dr. Hirsch told me that he would make sure they would not be interred in a place where people sympathetic to the terrorists could make a shrine of their bones. My understanding is that they were taken off U.S. soil. The four identified murderers and their unidentified criminal companions are not listed among the WTC dead, and no death certificates have been issued for any of them. But then again, none of their relatives have ever come forward to attempt to claim their bodies or request a death certificate. Let 'em try.

TWELVE

LONG BEFORE 9/11, my training and experience had taught me a great deal about the grieving process. I learned that mourners traverse through at least seven distinct phases, some of whose names have made their way into popular culture; today, most people are aware of the existence of the grieving phases of anger, bargaining, denial, and acceptance and are aware that each is a step along the healing process. My training also taught me though that having this knowledge doesn't make it any easier for the mourner to take those steps.

That is why nearly every religion, ethnicity, race, and social stratum creates complex rituals surrounding a member's death to provide structure and to ease the transitions through the stages of mourning. Wakes, funerals, memorial services, headstone unveilings, the Jewish post-burial ritual of sitting *shiva*, funeral masses, and the like are all examples of such death rituals. The rituals are so pervasive in our society that even non-relatives who have in some way been involved in a person's life expect to participate in the rites observed when he or she dies.

Normally, even when a family member's demise is sudden and violent, surviving relatives and friends derive benefit from rituals that help people to mourn and then to move on. But the WTC families were robbed of these normal rituals. For all those many survivors, it was as though their loved ones had simply left home one day bound for the Twin Towers and simply never returned, not even as a body to be buried or cremated. These families could not attend wakes for their son or daughter, or sit *shiva,* or take part in funerals, cemetery visits, or any of the social rituals that might have helped them make the transitions to a life after mourning.

The nature of these deaths, coupled with the absence of traditions designed to help families cope, led directly to the fifth major task the Incident Command Center handled: the development of a unit to interact with the victims' families, both at OCME headquarters and at the Family Assistance Center. Through our regular (non-WTC) case load, we were already dealing with the families of the more than twenty-four thousand dead each year, so we were well practiced in interacting with a decedent's next of kin. The WTC families, however, presented challenges related to the unique nature of their grieving processes.

I hate the word *closure* and try never to use it. My experience at OCME taught me that there really is no such thing. The notion of closure is almost insulting—you cannot tell a parent who just lost a child, "Hey, don't worry, you'll get over it." The wound of the death of a close relative or friend never completely heals; there is always a scar. We do, however, *transition* through the various phases of the healing process. The WTC families' unique situation was created in part by the prolonged process of the extrication and identification of the remains. It meant that months or even years might pass before their loved one was found, if ever. To make matters worse, the families were grieving under the harsh glare of the brightest media spotlight imaginable. Every reference to the WTC seen on television, heard on the radio, or read in newspapers, magazines, and web pages was like a dagger in the hearts of these families. They had no respite, no escape from being reminded of their loved one's death in the tragedy. As a result, many families kept spinning in an endless circle of grief, unable to break out of it and move on.

Their unending grief, in turn, placed a great deal of stress on the OCME employees who were interacting with them. In our regular, day-to-day work, OCME functions more like an ER than any other institution of medical care in that we tend not to have prolonged relationships with the families with whom we interact. In most instances, we meet the "patient's" family once and likely never again.

From the immediate aftermath of the attacks onward, we could see that our relationship with the WTC families would entail interacting with them repeatedly. In doing so, we would inevitably develop relationships with them that would interfere with an OCME employee's normal defense mechanisms for dealing with grieving individuals. It became difficult to keep a professional shell in place when the decedent's family member that you're talking to has become a dear friend.

We quickly realized that both OCME and the WTC families needed a special unit to handle this unique interaction. Having already seen quite a few WTC families at OCME headquarters, we understood that this was not a suitable place for repeated interactions. Moreover, our agency was not the only city or federal agency that needed to interact with the families. In was in this spirit that we set up the Family Assistance Center to appropriately house us as well as police, relief agencies, the Social Security agency, and nongovernmental organizations like the Red Cross. Because those agencies would be in residence there, the Family Assistance Center would also be able to help other New Yorkers—those who had not lost family members but were seeking assistance; for instance, people displaced when the collapse of the Towers destroyed or rendered their homes uninhabitable, and people whose businesses had been wiped out, throwing them and all of their employees out of work.

The Family Assistance Center was initially established across the street from the OCME office in an auditorium inside New York University Medical Center. It moved shortly to larger quarters at the Lexington Avenue National Guard Armory, a few blocks away. When that venue also proved not capacious enough, it was moved to Pier 94, which juts out into the Hudson River on Manhattan's West Side at Fifty-Seventh Street. Pier 92, next door, held the Emergency Operations Center, the headquarters for all the governmental organizations at work on the WTC disaster. Once situated at Pier 94, the Family Assistance Center really began to function seamlessly, as New Yorkers began to stream through the tight entrance security by the thousands.

I must admit that while I cared a great deal about the devastating ripple effect the attacks had created among those who had lost residences or businesses, my focus was on people who had lost a family member. As the person responsible for the Incident Command Center and the identification process, I quickly became the main person interacting with the families regarding OCME's identification of the victims. Meetings with the families were of two types. The easier ones, it may surprise you to learn, were those in which I told families that we had *not yet* identified their loved one but were working on it. Much more difficult were the interviews that followed a positive identification.

The "not-yet" interviews were easier but could not by any stretch of the imagination be considered *easy*. One such interview was particularly tough for me, because I had to tell the widow of my dear friend Jeffery Weiner, the assistant cantor of my synagogue, that we would probably never find any remains or identify anything of her husband. It was about a month after the attacks when Heidi Weiner came to see me at the office. Jeff had worked for Marsh & McLennan, and his office was on the north side of Tower One on the ninety-fourth floor. The nose of the plane had likely come through his office window. I wanted more than anything in the world to tell Heidi that we would absolutely find him, that I would work around the clock, move heaven and earth, and not rest until we did, but I couldn't in all honesty tell her that. Instead, during that interview in late October—the first time I had seen her since the disaster—I cautioned her that the overwhelming likelihood was that Jeff's remains would never be identified. A human body, I told her, can be fully cremated at 1,600 degrees Fahrenheit in as little as forty minutes. This was a month after the disaster, and the fires were still burning at the WTC (and would continue to burn for months more). That interview was agonizing for both of us.

I did hundreds of such "not-yet" interviews, many of them with foreign nationals who had flown into New York from as far away as Japan and Australia hoping to claim the bodies of their loved ones, and who felt they had to stay here until he or she had been identified and the remains released to them. The "not-yet" interviews were the easier ones because the information that I had to impart was straightforward:

"We have *not yet* identified him, but we're working on it, and we'll tell you the second that we've made the identification." As with Heidi Weiner, the families by and large understood the difficulties involved in making identifications under these extraordinary circumstances and were for the most part content to know that we were trying as hard as we could to identify the victims.

I say for the most part, because thanks to television, not every family came in to our office with realistic ideas of what we were able to do. I recall one interview with an elderly woman who wished to know why our efforts to identify her son were taking so long. She querulously pointed out that on a recent episode of the television show *CSI*, a "forensic scientist" had been able to obtain DNA results from a dead body in a matter of minutes. The hero just put in the sample, pushed a button, and out popped the identification, complete with a very nice photo of the victim. Why, she demanded, did we not have such a machine? Was it for lack of money?

I resisted the impulse to tell her that the same prop "DNA machine" would probably be used to make coffee in a later *CSI* episode. Instead I reassured her, as I did with countless other families, that OCME was in fact receiving adequate financial support for its WTC operations—which was true at least in that first year of operations— and that we had access to all the best computer equipment and programmers available. I explained, however, that obtaining DNA from severely damaged remains was a slow, laborious process, and even though the best minds in the country were working on the problem, it was going to take a long time before all the possible identifications could be made.

As time went on, I was able to become more optimistic with the families to whom I had to say, "not yet." With each passing week, our ability to identify remains was growing. When the Victim Identification Profile information sheets were all finally entered into the computer, we all received a collective boost; when our new DNA-matching software program came on line, another boost. And, of course, our own learning curve was steeply increasing with each passing day. All of these things added to the hope that many more victims would be identified than the two to three hundred we had initially (and privately) thought that we would be able to positively identify.

The other sort of family interviews, those that occurred when a decedent had been identified, were much more emotionally difficult for the families and for me. "We're about to have the most difficult conversation you'll ever have," I would often say as I began to speak with them and go on to explain precisely what remains had been found, in what condition, and what OCME had done to identify the person from whom the remains had come. For these individuals, this was the first confirmation that their loved one was definitively dead and had been identified. Although expected, it was nonetheless a blow because it eliminated any possibility that their loved one might be alive somewhere in a hospital. Although unrealistic, this hope reflected a universal wish. In 2005, after a WTC victim's remains were identified, a family member told a reporter, "Well, that's it, I guess he's not running around New Jersey somewhere with amnesia. I guess he really is dead." We received many, many similar responses during the course of the WTC identification effort.

On the other hand, a great many family members, after receiving notification that their loved ones had been found, sagged with relief, because at least now they knew. During the difficult times at OCME, this type of response served to bolster our conviction that we were doing crucial work. Families yearned for positive identification, if only so they could have certainty about the death and something to bury. As one firefighter's widow expressed it to a reporter, in a sentiment I heard in a thousand variations from grieving relatives, "If he's not laid to rest, it's like he never was. I want something that marks that he was alive. It makes him real. It says he was."

Some families only wanted the reassurance, in our interviews with them, that we had made a definite, absolutely positive identification—that, and no more. Other families wanted to know precisely what we had done, what body parts we'd had to work with, what condition they were in, and where and when the parts were found. These latter families were personified for me by the relatives of James Cartier. James was twenty-six at the time he died, a newly minted member of the electricians' union, and he had been working at the WTC only a few months before the attacks. He was the youngest of six siblings, and his close-knit family became very active in a group dedicated to helping other families through the tragedy. When at last we identified some of James' remains, two of his brothers showed up to claim him. Michael Cartier donned a pair of gloves and held and cradled his brother's remains. It was as touching a scene as I've ever witnessed.

Not every family had the Cartiers' courage to touch the remains of their loved ones, but many families did ask to see the remains. We at OCME did not encourage this, because many of the remains were relatively small fragments, not even recognizable as human let alone as someone's sibling, parent, child, or spouse. If a family asked to see the remains, we first showed them the Polaroid photos that we kept in each decedent's folder. Most people were content with that. If they still insisted on personally viewing the remains we would suggest that they do so at the funeral home. Only as a last resort would we take the family down to Memorial Park and show them the actual remains.

To manage the families' often unrealistic expectations of what their loved one's remains looked like, I was often forced into offering long, graphic descriptions of the effects on the remains of decomposition and of the terrible forces unleashed in the collapse of the WTC buildings. I did so to convince family members that they would not recognize the piece of burned or decomposed flesh that we had identified. Early on, during an interview with a family that was having a particularly hard time picturing what decomposition does to a body, I hit upon a useful simile: I asked the family to imagine they had put a banana on a windowsill in September. What did they think it would look like if they came back in December?

"Did my loved one suffer?" "Was my loved one among the jumpers?" "Was my loved one burned to death?" Frequently, during the positive-identification interviews, I was asked one or more of these three questions that tore at the hearts and minds of all the families. In answer to the first question, I could provide some comforting information. Each of the towers collapsed in somewhere between six and nine seconds. That meant that each floor came crashing down on the next in a microsecond. Which meant, in turn, that death came to their loved one suddenly, like the turning out of a light switch—and the likelihood was that the loved one did not really suffer at all. No one "rode down" with the buildings. If a person was on the eightieth floor, he or she was killed the instant that the eighty-first floor came down on them. By the time the eightieth floor hit the seventy-ninth floor, the person was long dead.

I tried carefully to stay away from discussing an area about which we had very little information: whether their loved one might have been injured during the initial attack and then had lain wounded and suffering until the building fell, killing him or her. I was not always able to avoid discussing such possibilities, and when pressed I would say that while I was sure that some few unfortunate souls were thusly injured and trapped, forensic evidence showed that the vast majority of victims were not injured severely or even at all until the buildings fell down, killing them instantly. We knew this because examination of the remains had not revealed many instances of vital reaction to trauma. Vital reaction is living tissue's response to an injury. Your hand swells quickly if it is hit by a hammer, and blisters with equal rapidity if burned by hot oil in the kitchen. The absence of blistering, bleeding into fractures, or inflammation that we would have seen had the living tissue been badly injured before death helped us at OCME to conclude that the awful trauma we were seeing in the remains occurred *at the time of death.*

Along with questions about possible physical injury of victims trapped in the towers waiting to die, came queries about the psychological torture the situation must have inflicted on its victims. I learned from family members who had been "fortunate" enough to have a final conversation with a trapped victim that the victims had been calm and accepted their fate. Though hearing of such conversations always cut through my defenses and caused me to choke up, I was able to use this information about the psychological calm of the victims to comfort other families who had not been "fortunate" enough to speak to their loved ones in the moments before they perished and say good-bye.

To the other two questions—whether a loved one jumped or had burned to death—my answers were less definitive. We couldn't know from examining the remains if any particular person was among the jumpers, because when the buildings collapsed, they collapsed on top of anyone who might have jumped earlier, crushing them as thoroughly as it did those who had remained inside. Similarly, we couldn't say whether a particular person burned to death because all the charred remains had been subjected to the high-intensity fires of the burning buildings, which burned long after the person had died. All I could say to comfort families about this last matter was that even in regular house fires, most victims don't burn to death. Smoke kills people long before flames do, and smoke inhalation is actually not all that bad a way to go when compared to burning to death.

Astonishingly, despite the pain these conversations must have caused, many families told me during the post-identification interview that they considered themselves lucky. This thought was perfectly put to me by Edie Lutnick, who lost her brother Gary Lutnick: "I am the lucky of the unlucky," she told me sadly, because at least she had remains that had been positively identified. She added, "Who would ever have thought that to sit here and be told that you found a piece of my brother's body makes me one of the lucky ones?"

At times there was too much of that good luck. Another factor complicating the process was that remains were coming in every day, many of them *after* we had already identified earlier fragments of the body from which they had come and had previously notified the relatives of the positive identification. This meant that we found ourselves repeatedly notifying families about additional remains, which caused problems. Early in the process, we identified the remains of a man and had the usual post-identification interview with his wife. We had no way of knowing at the time, but the man's body had been blown into countless fragments, not all of which were found together or identified at the same time. After the fifth time we called and told her that we'd found and identified yet another body part—sending her each time into a new spasm of grief—she asked us to stop. Couldn't we come up with a way to notify her *once* at the end of the process? Hers was a good question and—since we eventually identified over 250 fragments of her husband—one well worth finding an answer to. So we began to ask families, during the first notification session, to indicate their preferences and sign an "authorization of release" form, directing us as to if, when, and how often they wanted to be notified in the event we identified additional remains of their particular loved one.

This is the all-too-human story behind the creation of the Authorization to Release form. Some families chose to be notified every time additional remains were identified, some not at all, and some only at stated intervals. The document also gave the families the opportunity to appoint a proxy, such as a funeral director, who could be notified in their stead.

One interesting consequence of the release form was that many families chose to never be notified of additional remains. Thus there are plenty of identified but unclaimed body parts at OCME that will eventually find a resting place in the permanent memorial along with the remains that will never be identified.

Paroxysms of grief took place in front of me, and I was not immune to them. Sometimes I teared up as the family did. More often I did not. I was gentle, compassionate, brutally honest, vague, or direct in proportion to what I sensed the family wanted from me. I was always sincere—the families sensed that—but functioned as though I had a valve on my emotions, calibrating the opening in reaction to what I perceived the family's needs to be in the moment. Some needed the valve to be wide open, for me to empathize completely with them, others needed it mostly closed, for me to hold on to my reserve so that they could let go of theirs. Sometimes, though rarely, the families and I even laughed together. Once, a widow asked me to show her exactly where her husband's remains had been found. I took out the grid map of Ground Zero and began to point to the various places at which the six fragments of his remains had been found. To my horror, the widow started giggling during the explanation, and then I became really worried as she broke out into peals of uncontrollable laughter. Initially taken aback, I then started to feel the hysteria build up inside of me, and after a few moments more I gave up trying to keep a straight face and joined her in laughing at the absurdity of our conversation. "He never did *anything* the easy way, that man of mine," she said to me. "This is so typical of him: dying, and I can't even get his body back in one piece!"

Even in that interview, the pain and grief came through, as they did more openly in virtually every interview that I did; yet during the time that I conducted hundreds of those interviews, I bore it all as stoically as possible. Today, though, recalling the family suffering those interviews entailed, I feel the weight of emotion more heavily than I did then, perhaps because now I no longer have to struggle to preserve myself for the work of seeing the next family, and the next, and the next. Recalling these interviews and their extreme emotionality now, I move slowly, as though under a great weight, and each step feels enormously difficult to take.

When the identification process got into full swing, which enlarged the number of families waiting to be told that their loved one's remains had been identified, other people in the office jumped into the family counseling task. Katie Sullivan was one. Jimmy Meyers and Tammie Natali, two of the twenty new MLIs that OCME hired after 9/11, also became a mainstay of the family interview room. As with others who counseled the families, Jimmy, Tammie, and Katie also burned out after a while. These interviews could not be done day in and day out for a prolonged period, while remaining sane and unaffected.

Dr. Hirsch sometimes saw families—those who would not be satisfied with hearing the news from a lower-ranked official. He invariably had me in the room during these interviews to explain in detail what we had found, how we'd identified the remains, and so on. That arrangement was fine with me; Dr. Hirsch had a much larger and a different responsibility than I did and needed to keep his attention focused on those larger matters.

Responding to the families' increasing demand for information about our efforts, we began to offer once-a-week tours of the DNA lab and other parts of the OCME facility to families who were waiting but whose loved ones had not yet been identified. Hundreds of grieving relatives took those tours, and I hope they were comforted by the sight of dedicated public servants working tirelessly to help them.

At my suggestion, we issued photo identification cards to the family members, which bore their name and the RM case number of the relative they lost, against a background of an American flag. These ID cards were later adopted by the city as the official form of identification for WTC families, accepted at all venues for the families, such as the Family Assistance Center, the temporary memorials, and the chapels.

By the end of October 2001, organizations of families had formed—of civilian families, that is. The family counseling units of the fire and police departments had long histories of dealing with families of service members who had died in the line of duty, and were well versed in such counseling. Although the death toll from WTC was on a vastly bigger scale than the uniformed services had ever had to deal with, their organization was such that the counseling units were relatively effective in helping their bereaved families. Since the majority of the victims had not been police officers or firefighters, this left the families of the civilian victims without a central organization representing them.

To Mayor Rudolph Giuliani's everlasting credit, he began to meet weekly with these nascent civilian family organizations and their members. He would call in representatives from the NYPD, FDNY, the property clerk's office, the Community Assistance Unit, and OCME and we'd report on our progress to the families and take questions. Those meetings started before the end of September, held at City Hall, usually in a room on the second floor called the Committee of the Whole. They were awesome experiences. I had previously been in a few smaller meetings with the mayor and some of the victims' families, and during them I was repeatedly moved by the warmth and gentleness with which Giuliani treated the families. The mayor made time for them and listened to them, sometimes receiving incredible abuse in the process but responding calmly and respectfully no matter how outrageous the attack.

In the larger meetings with the families, which featured officials of many agencies, Dr. Hirsch attended the first few, accompanied by Dr.

Robert Shaler, head of the DNA lab, and me. Later Bob and I became the only OCME representatives at most of the meetings. By the end of November 2001, the family meetings at City Hall began to be held more intermittently, but OCME continued to meet with the families' groups at our headquarters, first weekly and later biweekly. Dr. Hirsch would chair these meetings, and Bob Shaler and I would give the factual reports and take questions. Katie Sullivan also attended, and as she took on more and more responsibility, she eventually ran the show, scheduling the meetings, setting the agenda, preparing handouts, and delivering updates to the families.

Almost from the outset of the meetings, we began to treat these family groups as though they were our board of directors to whom we needed to report on how we were conducting our business. Nothing in our charter mandated or suggested that we do this, but compassion and integrity demanded it. Some family members who regularly attended those meetings became friends of ours. Since the meetings were often held late in the evening, not commencing until 7:00 P.M. or 8:00 P.M., beforehand, when Bob, Katie, and I were grabbing a bite to eat, more often than not we would be joined by one or more of the family members.

Among the more memorable was John Cartier, elder brother of James, the young electrician I mentioned earlier. John, a tradesman himself and also a biker, would pull up on his Harley Davidson motorcycle with its huge handlebars, park it outside the restaurant, and plop down at the table with us. To other diners, we must have made quite an interesting table, John in his biker's vest, bandanna, and ponytail, and Bob and me in our business attire. We didn't think it incongruous because John had become our brother.

After dinner we'd troop back to headquarters for meetings that generally lasted about an hour. A tradition we developed was for us at OCME to bring to each family meeting an individual whom the families had not yet met but who was working hard on their behalf—and whom we'd jokingly call "tonight's exhibit." One of the first such individuals we brought (she quickly became a regular attendee) was Amy Mundorff, one of the great unsung heroes of the WTC identification effort.

Amy is a short woman, but her air of competency and authoritative personality make her seem much taller. A forensic anthropologist, she played a critical role in the WTC identification effort. From manning the triage station down in the remains receiving area, to helping me conceptualize the big picture of the identification effort, to identifying victims from their bones, she took part in every aspect of OCME's response. In a few instances, during the identification process, I disagreed with her findings and, being the boss, did it my way—but I soon learned not to. Each time, without fail, in her area of expertise she was proven correct. So good was her record in this regard that when her identification based on bone fragments conflicted with an identification based on DNA, I learned to go with Amy's identification. She asserted that in the chaos of the debris, remains simply *had* to have become comingled, and so, no matter how carefully we obtained DNA samples, if the samples were from soft tissues there was a high risk of contaminated results. It was Amy who first championed the idea of sampling bones for DNA, whenever possible, simply because they were less likely to be contaminated.

Which is not to say that bones could always be trusted, either. The reason lay in how they were collected and delivered to us, a problem which Amy also brought to our attention. One day the remains of a firefighter were brought in, essentially some bones in bunker gear, the supertough turnout clothing worn in the field by FDNY personnel. Her expert eye detected that there were two left femurs (thighbones) in the bunker pants. As this was not the first time something like this had happened, Amy deduced—correctly, it turned out—that when recovery workers found bunker gear at the site, they were stuffing into that gear any other bones found in the immediate vicinity. Of course, the recovery workers were not trying to sabotage the identification effort, but were simply operating on the mistaken assumption that those remains must belong to the same firefighter as the remains in the bunker gear. We learned to treat all bones found inside of clothing as separate, individual remains unless the bones were clearly attached to each other by soft tissue.

Another "exhibit" who we were proud to bring to a family meeting, and one of the most important WTC volunteers to rotate through our office, was Tom Shepardson, founder and sparkplug of DMORT. Tom was of average height and appearance; in his fifties, he appeared younger and more slender than most of those his age. At first glance, you would have guessed that he was a farmer, not a funeral director from Schenectady, New York, let alone the most experienced mass-disaster expert in the United States. Though he may not have looked the part, he was. He had come up with the idea for DMORT in the early 1980s and started it as a committee of the National Funeral Directors Association. By sheer force of will, he managed to get the group affiliated with the federal government's Department of Health and Human Services (DHHS). In 1992 the DHHS created ten volunteer DMORT teams in as many regions spread across the country. You name the large-scale disaster, Tom had been there—air crashes from Alaska to Alabama, floods, tornadoes, and the 1995 bombing of the federal building in Oklahoma City. Tom and DMORT knew more about large-scale disasters and mass fatalities than any other group in the United States.

In the wake of the WTC attacks, Tom came to New York City, stayed for weeks at a time, and returned again and again for months, bringing with him hundreds of volunteers. The WTC disaster was no simple task, either for Tom or for the individual funeral directors and other DMORT volunteers. One gentleman from Waltham, Massachusetts, a second-generation funeral director, wrote an article about the mental toll of the task. Deployed by DMORT, he had stayed in New York for several weeks working on it, but was then, in his own words, "emotionally exhausted" by the large-scale carnage of the disaster, and had to go home "to recharge his batteries." When Tom wasn't in New York, he didn't go home; rather, he went to the site of the other plane that was crashed into a field in Pennsylvania. His efforts were an inspiration to me and many others, helping us to perform at the upper limits of our abilities and our physical and mental capacities for long periods of time.

I am sad to report that Tom Shepardson died suddenly, on February 18, 2003, in Schenectady, New York. In a press release issued the next day, Health and Human Services Secretary Tommy G. Thompson said, "As a volunteer, Tom's efforts to add mortuary affairs and forensic experts to the National Disaster Medical System brought comfort and peace of mind to thousands of families. The identification of victims and proper treatment of their remains is Tom's lasting legacy. He will be truly missed by not only everyone in the DMORT program but also the entire National Disaster Medical System."

I am very proud to have worked alongside a true American hero, shared a few meals with him, and called him a friend.

Ultimately, bringing in these "exhibits" for the families became a particularly effective tool for demonstrating to them that there were many people hard at work behind the scenes. When the families would feel that progress was slowing and that new developments were not being made, it was our hope that they would conjure these names and faces in their mind as a testament to the scores of men and women who worked around the clock to identify as many victims as possible.

THIRTEEN

NOVEMBER 12, 2001, a Monday, was celebrated as that year's Veterans' Day. As a New York City employee, I normally would have had the day off and might have been enjoying the last day of a three-day weekend, but since the attacks on the WTC, normal had gone out the window.

Bleary-eyed and exhausted after an all-nighter at the office, I had returned home for a few hours sleep, a shower, and a shave to try to clear the cobwebs before going back to the office. As I stepped out of the shower, I saw on my bedroom television set a local news channel's first images of a plane crash that had just occurred somewhere in the New York vicinity. The initial reports were vague as to whether the plane had gone down in New York City or in Nassau County, and as much as I hoped that everyone on board was all right, I simultaneously hoped the crash had taken place outside the city limits.

I suppose it must seem callous that my first reaction was a selfish desire that the crash would have occurred in someone else's jurisdiction, but I was fatigued and my shock at this new disaster unfolding only made me groan and mutter, "You've got to be kidding me!" After all that we had already been through, how much more could we take?

I was soon to find out, because within minutes I learned that the plane had indeed gone down within the New York City limits, crashing into a row of houses in Far Rockaway, a residential neighborhood in the southeast corner of Queens.

As with everyone else who heard about the disaster of American Airlines Flight 587, my first thought was that the terrorists had struck again. The answer to exactly what had made the plane go down was then unclear, but by the time I finished dressing, and the reports revealed that the plane was a jumbo jet—an Airbus 300—I understood that there would be hundreds dead, and that I must immediately return to the office.

While walking the six blocks to the office, I realized that my unsettled feeling entailed more than the adrenaline rush: The plane crash fed into some of my private fears that stemmed from the first plane crash that I had worked on as an MLI. It happened in the winter of 1992: US Air Flight 405 had tried to take off at LaGuardia Airport in the middle of a late winter storm, and instead slid off the runway into an icy Flushing Bay. The Fokker 28 jet broke apart as it slid, burst into flames, and finally came to rest in shallow water just off the end of the runway. There had been fifty-one people aboard, and twenty-eight died.

I was on duty that night, and when my two-way radio went off with news about the plane crash, I was in the Bronx at a homicide. Within moments I was pulled from that job and ordered back to OCME headquarters, there to meet up with other personnel and prepare to head to the airport. When I arrived at the office, Sergeant Mark Geffen, supervisor of the NYPD Missing Persons' detectives assigned to OCME's Manhattan office, was putting together our emergency field mortuary kit. We loaded it into the trunk of his unmarked police car and he and I, together with Dr. Hirsch and other staff members, headed to LaGuardia in two cars.

We expected that the airport would be in turmoil when we arrived, so Mark was continuously on his police radio, attempting to alert the Port Authority police (who run New York's two major airports) that we were en route and with the CME. Unfortunately his messages didn't get through, and we were held up for some time at the sealed-off gate while the Port Authority cops laboriously tried to confirm with their superiors that they could allow the Chief Medical Examiner of the city to enter the scene of a mass fatality.

While we were waiting in our cars, one of the Port Authority cops abruptly motioned us to pull over to the side, then hurried to open the gate and stepped back, windmilling his arm as he ushered an oncoming vehicle through. I craned my neck to see who it was, certain from the cop's reception that it must be the mayor or perhaps the president of the United States. Before I could see the vehicle I heard it, a clanging sound reminiscent of an antique fire truck. Finally it came into view as it barreled through the gate—the Red Cross coffee truck, driven by two adorable little old ladies in yellow slickers and large yellow fisherman's rain hats. Clearly, we would have gotten in more easily if we'd been masquerading as a Red Cross coffee team.

Eventually, the Port Authority cops decided that the Chief Medical Examiner of the city might be permitted in to deal with the dead. We were directed to a maintenance hangar where Airport Operations had set up an Incident Command Center and temporary morgue. There were already a number of bodies and body parts laid out on the floor, and the entire place was fouled with the pungent smell of jet fuel that had spilled into the water and permeated everything it touched—remains, luggage, clothes, airplane seats, and other debris. The fuel spill made things more difficult not only because it stung our eyes and nauseated us but also because of another effect that I would learn about during the next twelve hours. Shortly after arriving at the airport, I went to the crash site itself and helped recover remains. I found a severed hand with polish on the nails and brought it back to the hangar. Next morning, when we looked at the hand again, the nail polish was gone—blanched off by the jet fuel, which had also obliterated the writing on the toe tag that had accompanied the hand, and many of the other toe tags, thus making identification more difficult.

Working all night in that hangar, with the sickening smell of the jet fuel around me did more than just turn my stomach. The experience evidently seeped into my unconscious; thereafter, whenever I smelled jet fuel at an airport, I began to feel nauseous and panicky. To this day, I'm forced to will myself to suppress that panic to get on a plane. The first time it happened was about a year after the LaGuardia crash, as I was about to board a plane—at that very airport—on a trip out of town to deliver a talk about that very crash. Although I'd always been a fearless flyer, I hadn't flown since the crash, and my sudden panic symptoms surprised me. I forced myself onto the plane, took my seat, and concentrated on breathing. My training in medicine allowed me to understand what was happening to me, and although I knew my fear was irrational, I was nonetheless helpless to control it. I began to imagine what would happen if this plane, too, slipped off the runway or burst into flames; I imagined the passengers as they would look after they'd been torn apart or burned to death, even though, of course, if they were dead at that time, I would be also.

Fortunately, I was sitting alone when these thoughts came to me, or else I would have been terribly embarrassed. A flight attendant noticed my distress and asked, "Nervous flyer?" I blurted out to her that this was my first flight since working last year's plane crash. Without saying a word, she walked away and came back a few moments later with two little bottles of liquor and a glass with ice. I accepted them gratefully.

People always ask me whether I have nightmares, given all the horrible things to which I have been exposed over the years of working at OCME. My answer is, "No, never." I can't recall even a single bad dream or loss of sleep due to my work. So far, this terrible fear of flying has been the only real price for my years of exposure to traumatized human remains. Over time I've learned to manage it, and though I prefer being on large planes to small ones, I have even been able to board small commuter planes—most of the time without the little bottles.

Although twenty-eight people perished and I picked up a phobia of flying, there was something positive that came of the US Air plane that slid off the runway. From that incident, the aviation industry gained a new understanding of how important it was to have planes properly deiced before takeoff in frigid weather. This in turn led to new regulations, which have likely saved more than a few lives. As the Latin motto in the lobby of OCME suggests, the dead always have something to teach the living.

Weather though, did not appear to have played a role in the crash of American Airlines Flight 587, because November 12, 2001, was a clear day with temperatures around 50 degrees Fahrenheit. By the time I reached my office, I had sketched out a plan to deal with this new disaster as my work on the US Air crash equipped me to envision the work we at OCME would have to do on this far larger crash. Flight 587 had been en route from JFK Airport to the Dominican Republic when it crashed less than two minutes after takeoff. All 260 people aboard the plane were killed, along with 5 people on the ground, where parts of the plane landed. There were 9 people in the plane crew, and the 251 passengers included 5 unticketed infants who had been sitting on their parents' laps. Most of the victims on the plane, 180 of them, were Dominicans. Some of these were citizens of the island republic who were returning home, and some who lived in the several Dominican enclaves in New York City were going to the island as visitors. The regular Monday-morning flight was a popular one because it was one of the least expensive. This particular plane was packed because the fare on the flight was about to be raised, considerably, for the forthcoming Christmas season, and many people wanted to take advantage of the lower rate to return home or to visit relatives before the fare increase took effect.

Had the crash of Flight 587 preceded the events of 9/11, it would have been the largest disaster ever faced by OCME and setting up a system for identifying multiple deaths would have been a major challenge. But because the crash of Flight 587 occurred two months and a day after 9/11, this new disaster ended up feeling relatively routine. Even I was surprised by how well prepared we were to handle this new challenge.

By 11:30 A.M. on November 12, we had set up in the OCME mortuary a separate and segregated path for receiving the remains from the air crash, as well as a system to collect postmortem information. The segregated receiving area and the assignment of a Disaster Queens (DQ) number to each of the remains would ensure we would not mix up plane crash victims with the Disaster Manhattan (DM) WTC victims.

Upstairs in the conference room, we also got to work quickly. By 1:00 P.M., the WTC Incident Command Center was renamed the "WTC and Flight 587 ICC" and was ready for the plane crash victims. We had created an empty copy of the WTC database into which information on the crash victims could be put, had made a few critical modifications of the software, and on every computer in the Incident Command Center, a new icon on the screen displayed the logo of American Airlines. By 1:30 P.M.,we were so ready that we were all looking at each other, trying to figure out what we might have forgotten, since surely it could not have taken so little time to set up the entire identification process for a major air crash. In the two months since 9/11, we had grown so accustomed to mass fatality work on a colossal scale, and we had so many resources readily available, that Flight 587, horrible though it was in information-processing terms, simply felt like a little bump in the road.

Later that day I met with Office of Emergency Management Deputy Commissioner John Odormatt at the Jacob Javits Center, the largest conference facility in Manhattan, located not far from Pier 92 and the headquarters of the Emergency Operations Center. It was a good choice for the site of a Family Assistance Center to be devoted exclusively to victims of the plane crash. My assistant director of identifications at OCME had been born in the Dominican Republic, so I dispatched her to the Javits Center to establish and run the Family Assistance Center. By 2:00 P.M., we had the airplane's manifest, provided by American Airlines. This was an unusually quick response from an airline, but Tommy McFall, the leader of the American Airlines disaster-response team and a familiar figure at OCME since 9/11, was incredibly helpful. The passenger list showed that the plane's passengers also included people from Taiwan, France, and Israel; one passenger, we would later learn, had previously managed to escape alive from the WTC disaster.

All of this occurred before the first remains reached OCME at 3:30 P.M. on November 12. Not only were the remains from Flight 587 in much better shape than those we were working with from the WTC disaster, but with the passenger manifest in hand, the scope of this disaster shrank to become a "closed universe." Nevertheless, despite the relatively small number of victims, positive identification of all the victims was by no means an easy task, because the information that we were able to obtain on the victims, particularly on those who held Dominican citizenship, was a mess. It was astonishing to me, in the wake of 9/11 and the new security measures that it had mandated, how many people on Flight 587 had been traveling with "fuzzy" documentation.

For the next twenty-eight days, until we had identified every victim, I would go twice daily to the Family Assistance Center, from where OCME staffers would send me distress signals about the difficulties they were having in extracting information on which we could rely. Part of the problem was structural. Whole families had been traveling together and had perished, so there were no close surviving relatives who could give us precise information or DNA samples to help identify those victims. Complicating matters was the difficulty that stemmed from incorrect spellings of names. Members of one family spelled their name three different ways, which made for difficulties in labeling samples and proper identification.

A third problem, especially for our DNA lab, was that many of the Dominicans in our closed universe were related to one another. Some, we would later discover through DNA analysis, were related to one another differently than had been reported to us— for example, first cousins were actually half sisters. Some other "family" members were not even blood relatives. All these circumstances made managing DNA matches, and keeping reliable track of family relationships between the donor and the decedent, a complicated task. We sometimes had to make guesses about the right relationship; in several instances, these hunches were later verified by the DNA lab analysis.

Adding to OCME's difficulty in performing the identifications were the families' attitudes toward what had happened to their loved ones and toward our effort to make identifications, while returning bodies and body parts to them for burial. Perhaps it was the nature of the airline crash disaster; perhaps it was the families' belief that having the manifest and the bodies in hand should have made the identification process easy—whatever the reason, some families of Flight 587 victims, far more than the 9/11 families, were frustrated by our progress and by our inevitable mistakes. This led to interactions with many of the families that were often much more challenging than those with the WTC families.

One such exchange occurred a few days after the adult children of an elderly victim left with their mother's remains. A particularly difficult family, we were relieved to see them on their way. Later that week, while working with some DQ remains, Bob Shaler discovered that the number 587 had been typed into the computer in place of the number 578 for a particular piece of remains. It was an honest mistake, doubtless helped along by the fact that the flight number was 587, but the remain number should have been 578. Of course, as luck would have it, the mislabeled remain was among those that had been sent to the difficult family. Bob promptly called me to his office and informed me of the mistake. Though it's the sort of numeric mistake that happens every day in a bureaucracy, we knew at once that in this highly emotional situation, it would be painful for the family to accept.

We knew too, at least theoretically, that if we never said a word, no one would be the wiser. Tempting as staying silent was, it was not an option. No matter how large or small the error, once we'd discovered what had happened, Bob and I both knew that the family must be immediately informed. We were professionally and ethically obliged to do this and, if possible, to rectify the mistake so that all the families could be assured that we were not hiding mistakes of any kind. Only by acknowledging our errors could we expect the families to have confidence in the remainder of our work.

I found Tommy McFall from American Airlines, told him what happened, and that I had to speak with the family immediately. The airline's care team, stationed at OCME, was keeping track of every family's whereabouts. To my dismay, I learned that the entire family had gone to the Dominican Republic for the funeral of their mother. Tommy shrugged and said, "We [American Airlines] have a flight leaving in three hours; if you can get to the airport I will take care of the tickets." I told Dr. Hirsch what had happened and that I was going to the Caribbean to correct the error.

By late afternoon, I was in the Dominican Republic. Alerted to my mission by American Airlines representatives, the Dominican government had graciously agreed to furnish me with bodyguards, including a plainclothes officer and two uniformed and armed soldiers, for the duration of my stay. I was glad to have them with me.

After a runaround worthy of a *Keystone Kops* episode, we finally located the family in a hotel, and via several intermediaries, I made an appointment to go and see them. Through an interpreter also provided by the government, I told the family what had happened: We had correctly identified all the body parts of their mother except one, a hand, which we had erroneously included. I further explained that we needed to take that hand back. After hearing this news, a member of the family spit in my face. Other family members hustled him out of the room, though none apologized. After we got back on track, I explained that the hand, which belonged to another victim, would have to be exhumed and returned to our office so that we could process it properly and convey it to the family of the person to whom it had belonged. After some more shouting, reason prevailed, and twenty hours after I had touched down in the Dominican Republic, I was on a flight back to New York. The hand would eventually follow me back to the United States, but only after lengthy negotiations between U.S. and Dominican authorities, and between funeral directors in both locations.

Despite such minor setbacks, by December 12 our OCME team had identified all the victims of Flight 587—a record short time for identification in a mass-fatality disaster. Years later, the National Transportation Safety Board (NTSB) identified the cause of the crash as a combination of pilot error and an overly sensitive rudder-steering mechanism. Following in the wake of a larger aircraft, the plane had encountered turbulence, and the pilot overreacted to that turbulence with a violent rudder maneuver, tearing off the tail stabilizer and putting the plane into a dive from which it was unable to recover.

This explanation has not satisfied some of the victims' families as well as some aviation experts, and today, long after we determined who the victims were, the legal assessment of blame is still under way.

Late in November 2001, with the WTC effort well in hand and Flight 587 all but wrapped up, I traveled to London as OCME's representative to a memorial service at Westminster Abbey for the British victims of the WTC attacks. Her Majesty's government had invited members of NYPD, FDNY, and other city agencies who had been instrumental in the recovery and identification of British victims of 9/11 and had given us round-trip tickets and hotel rooms for several days. Former president George H. W. Bush was the official leader of the American delegation, and as we were preparing to go into the chapel, he spotted a pin on my lapel that had been given to me by a British friend to wear for the occasion. It was two flags, the British and American ones, side by side. President Bush admired the pin, said he ought to be wearing something like that. Of course I offered to exchange mine for the American flag pin he had in his lapel. We switched pins, and I became the proud owner of a pin that had graced the lapel of a former president.

While in London, I received a telephone call with the following message: "One of our ID mistakes is on the front page of the *New York Times*. Above the fold." I was on the next plane home. The identification effort had been going along as well as we could hope, with a goal of zero error. Unrealistic, perhaps, but nonetheless we were striving for perfection, and though we knew we'd made a few mistakes, we were trying to hold ourselves to an incredibly high standard. Though a significant mistake, the one that had me on that plane hadn't been our first. That first erroneous identification happened back in the second week of our work but wasn't caught until late in October. It entailed a partial torso that had arrived downstairs in the morgue with a portion of a white shirt still on it, and with a photo ID card in the pocket of that white shirt. We checked the antemortem folder of the man on the ID card; his family's description of what he had been wearing on 9/11 included the mention of a white shirt. This, we supposed, was a slam-dunk identification, and we labeled the remains by the name of the ID card's owner and gave them to that family for burial. Then in October, our DNA laboratory came up with bad news: the DNA from the torso and the DNA from a toothbrush used by the ID card holder did not match. They were from two different people.

By this time, the torso had been buried in South New Jersey.

I immediately informed Dr. Hirsch. If I hoped he would respond by picking up the phone and talking to the family himself, I was mistaken. "When are you going to tell the family?" he asked. "This afternoon," I answered. "And I'll go and see them."

Which I did, accompanied by two Port Authority police detectives; the remains I was about to take away from the family were those of a Port Authority employee. We had also taken the precaution of asking the family to meet us at their funeral home and requesting that the funeral director notify the family priest and ask him to be present when we got there. The funeral director graciously did as requested.

I walked into a room at the funeral home and found the family seated in chairs arranged in a semicircle around one single empty chair in the center. Taking a deep breath, I sat in the chair and began to talk to the family.

On the way down to South Jersey, I had tried to put myself in the family's shoes. Our call had alerted them to our visit, and they were no doubt expecting something dire and waiting for a city official to come and tell them that "the system" had screwed up the most important thing in their lives at that moment—their attempt to make the transition from mourning to getting on with their lives.

My attitude was apologetic, humble, and straightforward.

Many years earlier, Dr. Hirsch had given me important guidance in matters of mistakes. "Perfect is not in our job description," he'd said, "but honesty is." The key was complete honesty and candor—more candor, I suspect, than many families might expect in such circumstances. I told this family in South Jersey that we had made a mistake—not that "a mistake had been made," but that *we* had done it, and we were owning up to it—and I explained how it had been made. Perhaps naively, we had presumed that the ID card belonged with the torso, and had made a positive identification too fast, not waiting for the DNA evidence to confirm the identification. Now the DNA evidence had shown that the identification had been in error.

To this day, no one can be certain exactly what happened to produce the odd situation of an ID belonging to one person showing up in someone else's pocket. My guess is that the owner of the white shirt survived the initial hit of the airplane, but that some of his colleagues did not; the white-shirted man probably picked up the ID of a coworker, thinking he would take it outside as evidence for that family of their loved one's death, and then a little while later he himself died with it in his pocket. We later began to notice just such things among the remains: One man was found wearing another's backpack. Several people had the wallets of others in their pockets. Another dead man came in with five cell phones in his body bag, and we had quite a time trying to figure out which of those, if any, was his. I don't think any of these folks were stealing. Rather, I firmly believe that in the interval between the planes hitting and the towers collapsing, the survivors of the initial attack attempted to gather identifying objects from their colleagues who were already dead. September 11 is like an onion: the more layers you peel away, the more heroism you find.

Considering how painful the news that I brought to this South Jersey family was, they took it very well. After all they had been through, losing their son, their brother, here I was about to take away the one comfort they had retained, the knowledge that they had given him a proper burial. That family displayed stunning graciousness to me under the most trying of circumstances. Similarly, in the several other cases in which we made mistakes necessitating a dreaded pilgrimage to a devastated family, I was treated far better than I might have treated the authorities if the mistake had happened to my family or me. I came to believe that my good treatment at the hands of these families was due to their understanding that the error had not been born of neglect, but rather, had come about because we had not had all the facts in front of us when the identification was made.

Such families wanted to know that we were rectifying the mistake and that we were working to make sure that this sort of error would not happen again and afflict any other families. On that, at least, I could be somewhat reassuring. As in the case of all our mistakes, we tried to learn their lessons and perfect our system through such feedback. In this instance, we learned never to rush an identification on the basis of what we presumed (but had not yet confirmed) as conclusive evidence.

We are proud, justly proud I think, of being able to say that we never made the same mistake twice.

Still, a lot of damage followed from our occasional mistakes. One young widow was distraught. She had been left with three small children—and no income, since the breadwinner was now gone—and had been taking the children to the grave of their father, every week, so they could at least have some contact with him. Now even that modest consolation was to be taken from her and the children. How could she explain to them that their father was not only not alive but not in that grave any more? The young widow swore me to secrecy and did not tell the rest of her family that we had retrieved the remains. She continued to take her children to a grave—now an empty one—to help them grieve. Mercifully, about a year later, we did identify (correctly) her husband and gave the remains to her. She had them buried in the grave, without the children's knowledge. I learned from subsequent conversations with her that this final burial eased some of her immense burden.

On the whole, though, our error rate was extremely low, well under a half percent, and many of the mistakes we made were caught in-house and rectified before they could lead to false identifications and remains being released to the wrong family.

Another early mistake we didn't catch was the result of the mislabeling of a toothbrush. Initially we matched the DNA extracted from a toothbrush to the remains and released the remains for burial. Still later, we learned from next-of-kin DNA testing that the DNA of the remains did not match the family's DNA and had to recall the remains. The only conceivable explanation for the mismatch (after confirming that the decedent had not been adopted) was that the toothbrush had been mislabeled. It must have been given to us by a different family and somehow had ended up with the wrong case number and family name. Now we had a perfectly good identification for some remains that were sitting around with no family to go home to, and we had an "orphan" toothbrush without proper pedigree. In plain English, we hadn't the foggiest idea whose toothbrush it was. In this and in every instance in which a mistake was made, I found myself surprised that Dr. Hirsch never made any personal attempt to reach out to the families, choosing instead to cede that responsibility to me.

One case that was particularly difficult to handle on my own was one of the worst identification mistakes we made and the one that became the basis for the story on the front page of the *New York Times*. As noted earlier, FDNY and other uniformed services were fantastic about bringing in the remains of their own. In this instance, firefighters had brought in, and positively identified to us, the remains of a firefighter named Jose Guadalupe from Engine Company 54. The firefighters who brought in the remains were adamant that they belonged to Jose because FDNY had logged his last known location by radio transmission. He was the driver of the engine, and the remains had been found precisely where they had expected to find them.

Unfortunately, also among the missing was another firefighter from the same company named Christopher Santora. The two men had been close friends; Santora was a devoted "student" of Guadalupe, who was about fifteen years older. Santora mimicked his mentor in every way, down to wearing the same sort of herringbone-pattern gold chain, cutting his hair in the same style, and so on. Even more important was something unknown to them: Both men had a relatively rare bone defect, a bifurcated C-spine, a split in a high vertebra (the one that sticks out when you bend your neck forward). Only one in a hundred thousand people has this defect. In truth it is more an anomaly than a defect, in that it causes no symptoms or hindrance; some experts even describe it as a normal variant. Whatever the case, it is certainly uncommon, and the odds of it appearing twice within the same fire company are astronomically low.

As a result, we never even considered that the remains might belong to Santora. Pointed in the direction of Guadalupe by the firefighters who brought in the remains, we obtained an antemortem X-ray of Jose's neck, and sure enough there was the bifurcated C-spine. Combined with his jewelry and with the bunker gear he was wearing, this seemed to be another straightforward identification. But we did not realize, when we identified the remains as Guadalupe based on the FDNY's labeling and on the X-ray with the peculiarity, *that both men had the same defect.* Once again, DNA testing revealed our error; that happened when the "Guadalupe" remains matched samples taken from Santora's toothbrush. Unfortunately this did not occur until after the Guadalupe family had their funeral—which, ironically enough, was attended by the Santora family.

When I learned of the mistake, I informed Dr. Hirsch, as I did on every such occasion, and then contacted the fire department. FDNY

Chief of Operations Sal Cassano and I met up at a firehouse in Queens where we talked with the widow of Jose Guadalupe. I gently told her what had happened, and why, and that we were going to have to remove Santora's remains from her husband's grave to give them to the Santora family. I am unable to adequately describe to you how painful this was for her. I wasn't sure if she was grieving more for herself or for the pain that the Santora family was about to experience. Next, Sal and I headed to the Santora family residence and met with them. I did my best to explain what had happened and why; by the end of the day, we had a plan in place to retrieve Chris's remains from Jose's grave and return them to the correct family.

Thus, the problem had been handled, as best we could handle it before I went to London.

When I received the call in London, two thoughts entered my mind. First, that I must return home to deal with the public relations fallout from the *Times* story; and second, that it was no surprise that this particular mistake would be the one that found its way to the public, given the firefighters' zealousness in protecting their families and the families of their fallen comrades.

Identifying the remains was our primary task, especially after the bulk of the DX (judicial decree) death certificates had been issued. We wanted very much to be able to replace these with DM (physical remains) certificates and for many families, we eventually did. The total of DM certificates issued to families *after* we had already issued them DX certificates was a staggering 1,196, covering more than two-thirds of the victims whom we were able to identify positively.

Families wanted and needed to have burials and other funeral ceremonies that allowed them to complete their bereavement journeys, get on with their lives, and assimilate the shock of losing a loved one. That need was why we worked so hard, and so incessantly, at identifying the WTC victims.

It was a process that entailed both science and, if not exactly art, then certainly the use of our capacities for reasoning and imagination.

Although 853 victims would eventually be identified solely by DNA matches, in almost as many instances DNA was not sufficient by itself to make a match and had to be supplemented. Again, it's a matter of numbers. Some fifteen thousand of the twenty thousand remains we had received were small, and many of the small ones were in bad shape, which made identifications harder. About 40 percent of the identifications we made were what we called "composite IDs"—that is, they were the result of several fragmentary clues rather than of one big match. For these "multiple modalities" matches, to supplement the DNA we used dental X-rays, regular body X-rays, fingerprints, photos, tattoos, and "personal effects" (the objects found on or near the bodies).

The lay public usually thinks of the identification of a dead person in terms of how such activities are usually portrayed on television. The family comes in to the ME's office and a somber staff member pulls out one of the refrigerated drawers lining the walls of every television morgue, pulls back the sheet and the family bravely nods and says, "Yup, that's our Timmy." This depiction of an identification is not all that far from reality, aside from the fact that those individual-drawer refrigerators are not efficient and most jurisdictions no longer use them. Today we use multiple body, room-sized refrigerators and Polaroid pictures of decedents, showing the actual body only if the family absolutely insists.

We call that kind of in-the-morgue identification a "one-to-one" matching process. One family looks at one body, and answers one question: "Is it him or is it not him?"

There is also a "one-to-few" matching process, an example of which is that of a police lineup. The cops have a suspect in a crime, and they try to have him positively identified as the perpetrator, by having witnesses pick him out of a lineup that typically consists of a half-dozen people. A larger identification of this "one-to-few" type is what the FBI does with a fingerprint from a suspect. They put the print into the hopper, compare it to those on file, and it is either an exact match or no match at all. That kind of identification we call a "one-to-many" process.

Unfortunately, in the WTC disaster, we couldn't do either of these two matches, at least not initially. We had a universe of perhaps ten thousand people who were initially reported missing to be matched against some twenty thousand pieces of remains and maybe another thirty thousand exemplars and objects from the families. This is a "many-to-many" matching situation, of the sort that is impossible for a lone human mind to complete. Actually, it's even difficult for a computer—it could overload the computer's circuits.

So our task at OCME was to do everything we could to reduce this "many-to-many" to something like a "few-to-few."

Any adult walking down the street may have as many as a thousand points of potential identification, including eye color, eye position on face, hair length, hair color, hair texture, scars, teeth, dentures, jewelry, contact lenses, clothing, girth, shape, calluses, habitual gait and its resulting wear pattern on shoe soles and foot bones, as well as what he or she was carrying. A woman's shirt can be described by means of its color, size, style, designer label, position or number of buttons, and so on. Tattoos are marvelous for identification purposes, providing as many as a dozen or more unique points for comparison. The list of potential identification points goes on for pages and pages.

After our mistaken identification of the torso with the ID card, we decided that three points of matching information would be required for making an identification on any given remain. If we were unable to obtain three—for instance, if the remains were so small that we could not even verify which bone of a body it might have come from—we might still make a positive identification using DNA, but only after administrative review of all the evidence ensured that there was no conflicting data.

Fortunately, the bags of remains brought in to our office contained not only human flesh but also objects such as clothes, watches, rings, and other items that helped us narrow our search.

There were many propinquity clues—pieces found in proximity to one another. If you had a hand here, and six inches away there was a watch, there was a good chance that the hand and the watch had belonged to the same person, although you couldn't say so definitively without having a third clue that verified the first two. Such propinquity clues gave us a place to start. We called them hunches or vectors *toward* an identification and made sure to keep a wary eye out for any indication of conflicting data. If the slightest doubt surfaced that a particular identification wasn't 100 percent certain, it was shelved until more data and points could be obtained. Also, I had discovered to my chagrin that it was a lot easier to explain to a family why we had waited so long to make an identification, than to have to apologize to a family for having moved too quickly and having made an error.

So, more often than not, "composite identifications" were the rule. We had many partial fingerprints that by themselves were inconclusive as identifiers, but when combined with other clues, the partial print could edge us toward an identification. Eventually, we used more than forty different combinations of modalities to make identifications. We'd have a bit of DNA, a partial fingerprint, another partial hit from a fragment of teeth; each of these, by itself, would not suffice as a sole identifier, but if there were enough overlaps among all three, we could make a definitive match. Sometimes we'd need more than three clues to satisfy ourselves that our match was completely correct. We needed both "belts and suspenders," as Dr. Hirsch so often suggested.

One of our more esoteric identification modalities involved using X-rays of the feet of victims, as evaluated by Dr. Rock Positano, perhaps the only forensic podiatrist in the world. Rock heads the division of podiatric medicine at the Hospital for Special Surgery. Rock began his association with OCME in 1974 when as a high school student he convinced Dominic DiMaio, then the chief medical examiner, to allow him to intern one afternoon a week assisting and observing at autopsies. He went on to become the unofficial curator of the office's Black Museum, a collection of medical curios started by the fabled CME Milton Halperin. In 1989, as a freshly minted podiatrist, Rock convinced Dr. Hirsch that podiatry X-ray was a viable tool for body identification. Within a few months, he proved his mettle on a case of a female labor leader whose chopped up and burned body was found in a dumpster in Harlem; Rock was able to identify her, when no one else could, by comparing her remains to X-rays of her feet taken some time before she died.

Rock pointed out to us MLIs that mobsters never chop off a victim's foot at the ankle, because the interlocking web of twenty-six bones and many sinews at the ankle is too strong to be severed easily—and that feet left on the body can help provide a positive identification. Another interesting fact pointed out by Rock was that by the age of forty, 75 percent of all Americans will have had an X-ray of one or both feet.

During the 9/11 identification effort, Dr. Rock Positano's expertise, and the pool of available foot X-rays, proved invaluable, enabling him to identify a handful of victims that we might not have otherwise identified.

Once we were past what we at OCME referred to as the low-hanging fruit of the tree—the group of identifications that were fairly easy to make because of the size of the clues such as the 174 remains that were in the category of "whole body," the 55 remains that could be identified solely by means of dental X-rays, and the handful from foot X-rays—the task of identifications became much more difficult and therefore slower.

By December 2001, we no longer thought there were ten thousand or even six thousand victims, but we still believed our potential universe of victims could be as large as several thousand people. Shortly, we would narrow the list of the missing and the already-identified dead to 2,749 victims. Of these, we had only identified a few hundred. There were an awful lot of WTC victims waiting to be identified and many families anticipating our efforts.

Accordingly, the DNA effort loomed as even more important to the identification process. It was critical, in fact. Without DNA evidence, it was obvious to us at OCME that we would be able to identify only a few more of the victims. It had taken several months for a new software program for identifying DNA matches to be built (by an outside vendor, Gene Codes, in cooperation with OCME's DNA lab). The previous system, which had been developed for the FBI, couldn't handle the volume of remains and samples that we were dealing with. That was understandable because it had been developed to compare the DNA of one suspected felon with what was on file, and make a match. By December this system had identified 203 remains that belonged to 105 different people. On December 13, when the new Gene Codes system began work formally, that very day fifty-five new matches were made.

To our dismay, however, it turned out that this was about as far as either system could go, because we had a terrible problem. We discovered that the first collection effort of the antemortem DNA evidence was severely flawed. The errors appeared after Bob Shaler sent some of our DNA work to the New York State police crime lab at Albany for completion. When Albany showed us their results, though, it was clear that the samples taken from the families were inadequate for making the identifications.

DNA strands are made up of literally billions of individual bits of four chemical bases known by the letters A, T, G, and C. Because there are so many repeats, experts in matching DNA need to see unique patterns at thirteen different areas (loci) on the strand to make a match. If you can match, say, ten out of the thirteen loci, you can be pretty certain about your identification, but if you only have, say, six out of thirteen, you simply cannot make a positive identification.

Since much of the postmortem DNA—what we could get out of the body parts—was in bad shape, very degraded, it was even more important that the premortem DNA (brought to us on such things as toothbrushes, hairbrushes, razors) be in good shape. We also needed proper samples from the victim's relatives to add the necessary genetic information with which to make possible matches. Of the thousands of toothbrushes and other items collected, however, it turned out that hundreds had been mislabeled. In legal terms, their "provenance"— that is, where they came from—was unclear. Moreover, we lacked enough samples from family members to resolve the mystery of who, exactly, had used a particular brush. For example, if a brush contained the DNA of two people, when the family had thought it had only been used by the victim, whose was the second DNA? It could belong to a relative or, for that matter, to a visitor who had forgotten to bring along his or her own toothbrush and surreptitiously used one sitting in the bathroom instead. How could we know? In the absence of samples from all the people in the house, we were unable to figure out easily whose DNA was on that brush.

When we added up the figures, we were horrified: only 35 percent of the families had given us sufficient antemortem DNA samples. The police department team collecting the samples had simply done a lousy job of collecting the samples from the civilian victims' families, as well as from NYPD victims' families. The fire department had done not much better in collecting samples from its own service families—no surprise, since it had attempted to collect evidence from more than two hundred families of missing firefighters in a single day.

The decree from City Hall that placed the cops in charge of the effort to obtain DNA from victim families had turned into a debacle, and so had the effort by the firefighters to collect samples from two hundred families of firefighters. If only the cops and firefighters had not been so territorial and had permitted people with the proper medical and scientific training—people whose daily job it was to collect such samples—to have sat at the tables when they collected material from the families, many of these mistakes could have been avoided.

Mislabeling of hundreds of items was a calamity, but perhaps the worst things about the situation were the tremendous missed opportunities. In one instance, a foreign family had come in, from a great distance away, to give samples so their loved one could be identified. The cop taking the samples looked at the decedent's photo and at the family in front of him and decided that one brother looked almost exactly like the decedent and opted to take a DNA sample only from that brother, not from other members of the family. The cop's ignorance of how genetics works, and where DNA comes from, trampled that golden opportunity.

There are literally dozens of ways to get DNA samples from decedent's lives—but to obtain them you have to ask the right questions. For example: a medically savvy professional at the collection table might have asked a husband when his late wife had had her last menstrual period, and if by chance there might still be a used tampon in the garbage—such an object, if available, would have given us a very good sample of the decedent's DNA. Had there been a recent hospitalization during which the victim's blood was drawn? Perhaps a recent biopsy? Medically untrained cops didn't ask such questions, and few such samples were collected where surely more could have been. (I actually went to a dermatologist's office and picked up a skin biopsy that helped us identify a WTC victim.)

It was clear that we needed better samples, ones whose provenance was clear and direct. We would also need more next-of-kin samples from more family members.

At first we were uncertain how we should go about collecting these. To me, the answer was clear. "We'll have to issue a press release saying that we need more samples from the families and set up a hotline so that the families can call in and give them to us directly," I explained to Dr. Shaler and then to Dr. Hirsch. This way there would be no need or call for immediate finger-pointing because the job had been done improperly the first time. We would, of course, have to take some heat from the families for the delay, and for the problems caused by having to locate more items from the dead family member, as well as exemplars from the live ones, but as I saw it, we had no choice but to do this if we ever wanted to make the identifications.

While Dr. Hirsch understood the need and agreed about the remedy, he was initially reluctant about the path to obtaining the new samples through the use of a hotline. He thought we didn't have the personnel to staff it, twenty-four hours a day, seven days a week. I showed him, in detail, that we did, that it would not be difficult to set up six phone lines and have them staffed by MLIs and people from our DNA lab. Dr. Hirsch then agreed, and we began the process of setting up the hotlines and readying the press release.

After consultation with city hall, the press release went out right after New Year's, in January 2002, accompanied by articles in the newspapers and so on, asking the families to call us because we needed more samples. There was yelling. There was screaming. There was dismay. But very quickly these emotions yielded to a flood of calls from families to the hotline—calls that soon numbered in the thousands. We were soon obliged to ask peak-hour callers to call back at a less crowded hour—any time, in fact, since the hotline would be staffed twenty-four hours a day. By this method, we got a lot of good information at 2:00 A.M. as well as 2:00 P.M.

Some families who called in were asked to come down to our office, bearing more objects from the decedent and giving additional DNA samples. With other families, especially those who lived far from New York, we were able to send them a collection pack, together with explicit instructions on collecting and bagging their own samples, so that they could ship the required samples to us. For those families who lived abroad, the system was more complicated. Federal law prohibited commercial carriers without a special license from shipping biological materials across borders from any country into the United States. This led to our arranging for families from abroad to be able to "smuggle" in their samples via their countries' diplomatic pouches.

During this period, a woman showed up at the OCME office intent on seeing me. I was busy, and our staff kept her at bay for a while, but eventually I saw her because she insisted on talking only to the head of the identification program. In my office, with the door closed, she told me that her grown children were coming in to give DNA samples to help identify their father who had died in the WTC attacks. She instructed me that the samples should be taken but absolutely not used in the identification process, because the man her children thought of as their father was not their biological father. Her husband's sperm had been deficient, so they had used donated sperm and decided together never to tell their children. She was adamant that the children not find out at this inopportune moment that their father was not their biological parent. Of course we complied with her request. This case was not unique; other women came forward to confide that they had had an affair, or that there had been an adoption and the child who wanted to provide a DNA sample was not biologically the offspring of the deceased man.

The hotline eventually fielded around thirty thousand calls, and led to the collecting of ten thousand additional samples. The percentage of families giving us sufficient DNA to make identifications rose from 35 percent to more than 80 percent, and the samples led directly to the hundreds and hundreds of additional identifications we made over the course of the next several years. Among those were many of the 214 firefighters whose remains were eventually identified. As though to make up for its initially poor job collecting samples from the families, the FDNY discovered that it had even better samples for us, in the form of blood many of the firefighters had donated to a bone-marrow transplant organization, which had been stored away for later use. These pristine samples from the victims themselves helped us make many positive identifications of fallen firefighters.

I had never expected my friend Jeff Weiner's remains to be identified, because we had figured that the first plane had come right in the window of the North Tower office in which he and his colleagues at Marsh & McClennan had been working. In February 2002, however, a match was made between a small piece of bone found on the roof of WTC Building 5, more than a block away from the North Tower, and a sample of Jeff's DNA brought in by Jeff's widow, Heidi. Moreover, examination of Jeff's bone fragment revealed forensic evidence corroborating my suspicion that he had been caught in the initial impact of the plane and the subsequent explosion. What must also have happened—something I had not anticipated—was that the explosion hurled this fragment of Jeff's body out of the cataclysm and that it landed on the roof of a building far enough away from the epicenter to survive the collapse and the fires.

Identifying Jeff reinvigorated my own dedication to the task. With permission from Heidi Weiner, I used Jeff as an example in almost every "not-yet" interview I did, as proof that anything was possible and that no family should lose all hope.

The month of March comes in like a lion and goes out like a lamb, or so the saying goes, but that could also have described my physical and mental condition in early 2002. By March of that year, the WTC identification process was well under way, and a steady daily routine had developed in the Incident Command Center. At that point, we had identified hundreds of victims from thousands of body parts. I was still working sixteen-hour days, seven days a week, as March began, but by the end of the month, I found that the work was catching up with me, and I became ill. Just how ill I didn't even know at first—until one critical meeting approached, and I suddenly grew worried that I might not be able to attend it as the OCME representative.

The fire department had arranged for all the families of the fallen firefighters to meet in an auditorium on Staten Island, to be updated on the identifications process and have the opportunity to talk to city officials responsible for the recovery effort. Fire Department Operations Chief Sal Cassano, who had become a fast friend, had relayed an invitation to me from the newly appointed fire commissioner, Nick Scopetta, to join them on the podium, representing OCME and the identification effort.

Though I felt increasingly ill, I also felt I couldn't ask Dr. Hirsch to go in my place because he'd had such a negative experience at the first firefighter's family meeting that he swore he would never do it again. I understood why: when they got together, the FDNY families tended to show great hostility toward the city government. This greatly pained beleaguered city officials like Dr. Hirsch, who felt they were doing all they could but were nonetheless vilified.

In the weeks leading up to the firefighter families meeting, I began to develop night sweats, and eventually severe joint pain and crushing fatigue. The symptoms progressed to headaches, nausea, and finally, a pain on my left side that at times took my breath away. For years I had been a dedicated consumer of four or five daily cups of coffee, but now I developed a strange aversion to this happy addiction and felt even worse as I went into caffeine withdrawal. I dragged myself around the office until, one afternoon, Dr. Hirsch stopped me in the hallway and said, "Shiya, I've autopsied people who looked better than you do. Go home!"

Instead of going home, I went to see Sidney Stein, the best internist in New York City. My family doctor and a friend for many years, Sidney took some blood, sent me for a sonogram of my side, and commanded me to get some rest. I went home, but returned to work the very next day. Shortly, the diagnoses came back: a severe case of mononucleosis and an alarmingly enlarged spleen (the cause of the pain in my side).

On the day of the firefighter family meeting, I developed a temperature of 103 degrees Fahrenheit, along with mild encephalitis (brain swelling). I knew I had encephalitis because I'd begun experiencing the visual disturbances known as "Alice-in-Wonderland" phenomena. My field of vision was continuously rippled, as though someone had dropped a rock into a pool; the ripples would spread from the center of my visual field to the periphery, clear up, and then a few moments later begin again. I figured the encephalitis must have been mild, because I was still walking around and talking, but I wasn't sure how much longer I could do that. So I took Katie Sullivan with me to the meeting.

The event began with Nick Scoppeta introducing himself to the assembled family members and receiving a reception that was tepid at best. Next up were two French brothers who had produced a film about the fallen firefighters. The film was set to air on national television shortly, and the families were incensed that they had not been consulted. The filmmakers faced a very angry crowd. I was up next, and by the time the brothers finished, I was in a state of dread.

Perhaps it was the fever, perhaps the encephalitis, but for whatever reason I was preternaturally calm. I introduced myself, and within a few moments, I had the families' rapt attention. I spoke slowly and clearly (I don't think I could have spoken rapidly had my life depended on it), telling them that we were still trying to identify their loved ones, that we would continue to do so to the limits of our physical strength and the limits of science. Perhaps the mono made me appear so weary that the families perceived just how hard we were working. I can't explain why the families calmed down as I spoke, but it was surreal. As I finished speaking, they applauded, asked me questions, and warmly thanked me and OCME for the efforts we were making on their behalf. I felt like I was on death's door, but it was one of the best nights of my professional life.

On the way home, I realized that the calm I had artificially marshaled for the sake of the families had crept inside me—that I actually *was* calm. For the first time since 9/11, I was at peace. That peace birthed a revelation in me. We were doing all that we could and more, and a tough audience had recognized that. I couldn't go on killing myself, working all day every day without a break, not while I was battling my own illness. I had to slow down, to bring some balance into my life, or shortly I would burn out and be of no use to anyone.

FOURTEEN

BY EARLY APRIL 2002, I had recovered enough from my illness to start functioning properly again. To regain my equilibrium, I cut back on my insane hours, shifting some of the workload to Katie Sullivan and others. That didn't mean I altered my emphasis on compassionate care or on identifying the victims and bringing peace to their families. I remained devoted to the WTC identification effort and still gave every WTC family member I spoke with my cell phone number and let them know they were free to call me anytime, day or night.

Coinciding with the reduction in my hours, the overall OCME workload for WTC began to level off as the initial phase of the recovery work approached an end. The receiving area, for instance, was now open only sixteen hours a day instead of twenty-four. Through the late winter and early spring of 2002, the pace of arrival of new remains tapered off; by May it had essentially concluded. Shortly thereafter the Ground Zero site was officially closed, at least for the purposes of recovering remains.

In the task of cleaning up after the WTC tragedy, an important shift in emphasis had begun back on January 1, 2002, when Mike Bloomberg took office as mayor of New York City, replacing Rudy Giuliani, who was prevented by term limits from running for a fourth term. From my perspective, the change in administrations was striking. Giuliani and his team had concentrated, in the months after September 11, on recovery of the remains and on comforting the bereaved families. The Giuliani administrators also kept the city going, but anyone who was working for the city during that time will tell you that WTC and the victims' families were issue number one. The Bloomberg administration came in with new priorities. While it also pledged to recover, renew, and rebuild the city, its emphasis was on renewal and rebuilding.

The WTC families felt the difference keenly, and many of them complained bitterly to sympathetic ears at OCME. They saw the change, in part, as a matter of personal style; where Giuliani had been very warm and close to the families, Bloomberg's style was more managerial, more businesslike, more politely distanced. I believe that Giuliani's remarkable warmth and affection for the WTC survivors and victims' families can be traced to his own narrow escape from the falling Towers on September 11. Rudy Giuliani breathed in the dust at the site and barely escaped with his life; the experience seared him. Even today, his public statements since leaving office indicate his continued strong support for the WTC families.

In truth, this shift in styles and Bloomberg's emphasis on being an all-about-business mayor were not a bad thing. The city desperately needed that kind of management if it was going to pull itself out of the shock and sadness that threatened to overwhelm it. Businesses, particularly in the financial community, were pulling out of the city, or threatening to do so, and taking with them thousands of jobs. New York City was obviously at a major crossroads in its history, and I believed that Bloomberg was the right man to lead New York out of the tragedy and into the future.

Still, it was a shame that his style left many WTC family members feeling cast aside. Many of the families felt that the differences between the two mayors went beyond stylistic issues, and that the Bloomberg administration's agenda—for example, in the rebuilding at Ground Zero—was completely at odds with what the families wanted.

On the day in May 2002 when the recovery site was closed, a ceremony was held at Ground Zero. A piece of WTC steel, the last remaining in the pit, was symbolically brought out, draped in an enormous

American flag. Many of those who had played key roles, and some who were still actively involved in the recovery and identification effort, were invited to attend. Hundreds of us stood on "Tulley Road," the long ramp leading down into the pit of Ground Zero, and waited for the massive steel beam to be pulled past us. Bob Shaler, Tom Brondolo, and I, representing OCME, were on that ramp along with steelworkers, firefighters, cops, and governmental officials. Giuliani was there, standing alongside Mayor Bloomberg and Governor George Pataki; both of New York's senators and many other dignitaries and notables also lined the route. As the beam passed, we fell in line behind it and marched out of the pit, out of Ground Zero, and away from all that death.

As we strode for many blocks up the West Side Highway past throngs of applauding New Yorkers on the side of the route, it occurred to me that for most of the marchers behind that steel beam, this was indeed a closing ceremony. Their work was done, and the spectators seemed to feel that. No one was going to forget what happened at Ground Zero—as evidenced by so much effort having gone into organizing such a solemn, public ceremony, but it felt as though the city was getting up after a period of public mourning. We had veiled ourselves in black and we would never forget, but now we must carry on.

Still, for all the good intentions, I noticed in the facial expressions of Bob and Tom the same realization that I was reaching myself: for the New York City ME's office, and for all the victims' families still waiting for a loved one's remains to be brought home, this day's ceremony rang a little hollow. The families were not yet out of the pit at Ground Zero, so we couldn't be either.

Back at OCME, work continued as though there had never been a closing ceremony. The complex DNA-matching programs, and our relentless efforts to reach out to the families to collect more DNA samples, were finally beginning to pay off, but slowly. By the first anniversary of the WTC bombings, on September 11, 2002, only around five hundred of the nearly three thousand victims had been positively identified. I was too busy at OCME to attend that day's anniversary ceremonies at Ground Zero; hundreds of families of the WTC dead, both before and after those ceremonies downtown, wanted to visit the Memorial Park where the remains were being stored, and I remained at OCME to assist them.

Since October 2001, when we first made arrangements for families to come to OCME and visit the adjoining Memorial Park, thousands of WTC family members had done so, paying their respects under the tent where the remains were stored. Interacting with the families at that time, even for such a routine task as escorting them to the family room at Memorial Park, was always a delicate and difficult process.

Often, it was complicated by interfamilial tensions. One of the more troubling aspects of the aftermath of the WTC bombings was that many significant others of the dead, who were legally not members of their families, were being shunted aside by the "real" families. This didn't happen in every instance, but there were plenty of such difficult cases. Partners, lovers, even fiancés were ignored in the grieving—and in the process of deciding who would share in the funds donated to assist the victims' families. I saw fiancées shoved away by blood relatives, even prevented from knowing whether their beloved's remains had been identified.

One woman who had lost her son came in to our office for the sole purpose of ordering me not to divulge any information to her son's fiancée. "I always hated her," the mother said, "and if she thinks she's going to cash in on my son's death, she has another think coming!" In some instances, the biological family excluded the fiancée even though the wedding date had been only a few weeks away. Long-term roommates, lovers, and even common-law spouses were similarly treated, as though they had little claim to grief—and none at all to survivor benefits. In many cases, this treatment seemed to me unfair; common-law spouses did have some legal protection, but the bereaved survivor had to cope with proving and defending the relationship in addition to suffering the usual emotional stress of sudden loss of the spouse.

As time went on, and the monies available to the victim's relations, through the federal Victims Compensation Board, swelled to life-altering proportions, I sadly found that fractures began to develop even among blood relations. I suppose it's not surprising: big money has long been known to produce squabbling among surviving relatives.

The spectacular exceptions to the rule gave me hope and kept me going. I remember seeing a father-in-law-to-be in the lobby of our building, holding his son's fiancée, both of them crying. "A week from now," he said through his tears, "a piece of paper would have stated that this woman is my daughter. Well, I don't need a piece of paper to recognize my family. This *is* my daughter."

Family infighting depressed all of us who worked closely with the WTC families. Witnessing this inequality of treatment firsthand galvanized me to propose to my then-girlfriend, now wife, Jennifer. Deep down, I had always known I would ask her to marry me; I had loved her from the day I set eyes on her. With a divorce behind me, though, I had been unwilling to rush into marriage again.

Now, you don't have to work at OCME for very long to figure out that life is short and precious, and certainly by 2001, I had seen too much death not to know that. But my work in the wake of 9/11 gave me an even greater appreciation for the beauty of life, for what I once heard described as "the magic of an ordinary day." Caring for the families of thousands of young, dynamic professionals who had died way too early, and who were not that dissimilar to me, taught me that life was too precious to waste even a moment. I asked Jenn to marry me. Lucky me, she said yes, and we set a wedding date and place: in our synagogue, early 2003.

As my work on the WTC identification eased a bit, I made time for other endeavors. During my spare hours, after work, I sometimes watched television, and became a fan of the *Law & Order* series. A fellow congregant at my synagogue, Roz Weinman, was a producer on the show, and from time to time I would call her to grouse about a forensics absurdity that had crept into the writing. From time to time, she asked me for forensics advice on a script in development. Now with a bit more time on my hands, this relationship was formalized, and I became the forensics consultant to *Law & Order*. It was a pleasure to be able to use my forensics knowledge in such a fun and creative endeavor. I worked with the writers on script development, coming up with interesting story devices to kill people, and even more interesting ways for the detectives to figure out how the death occurred. As time went on, I also worked with the props people, set designers, and special effects artists to make the death scenes look more realistic and interesting. This made for some pretty entertaining conversations: "No, don't use a hatchet," I would tell them, "make it a hammer—less shattering of the skull." "After three months in a salt marsh, the skin falls off the body as you pick it up." Anyone who overheard my cell-phone conversations with the producers and writers must have wondered which I was—a professional hit man or a homicidal maniac.

Since *Law & Order* is shot entirely in New York City, I regularly visited the set and got to know some of the actors and actresses on the series. Leslie Hendrix, who plays Medical Examiner Rodgers, became a particular friend. And before Jerry Orbach passed away, I had the pleasure of spending time with him in his dressing room, listening together to the cantorial music we both loved.

As the months wore on, the number of identifications we were making began to dwindle, from a rate of about a hundred a month to twenty or thirty, and then to only a handful. For many victims, we had no dental X-rays or fingerprints, and in the case of smaller fragments, we had no clues at all. Moreover, the soft tissue on remains found later in the recovery effort was in even worse shape than on those remains uncovered earlier; the inevitable process of decomposition had caused the disintegration of scars, tattoos, and other potential identification clues.

By the spring of 2003, DNA had become our one remaining tool. Soon after that, even the straightforward DNA identifications began to thin out, so we started using composite DNA matches—that is, employing several different DNA technologies to make a single identification. The remains from which we were now attempting to wring out a few more identifications were so degraded that a single DNA identification method would not give us a match we could count on as

100 percent accurate. When two or three such methods were combined, however, the likelihood of an accurate match rose. One DNA matching technique was based on mitochondrial DNA; another was called "short tandem repeats" (STR); a third was a kinship-DNA match.

What we were doing, by combining these methods, was coming nearer to closing the universe of potential missing persons. One DNA test allowed us to reduce the number of possibilities for a match from the thousands of people on the missing lists to, say, 250 people. We'd then run additional DNA tests, further narrowing the possible number of victims. When we reached just one possibility, we'd have a match. More often than not, we could not do that. When we were left with several possibilities, we had to deem those remains unidentifiable.

The process was extremely labor intensive and time consuming, demanding that individual attention be paid to each remain and each DNA test by the scientists doing the testing, the anthropologists working with the remains, and the Incident Command Center staff who were putting all the information together. By the end of 2003, our rate of identifications was down to a trickle—a steady trickle, but no more then that.

Making identifications in this manner was a very expensive as well as a very time-consuming effort. Identifying the dead of the WTC disaster ultimately cost around $80 million for just OCME's share of the work, according to an estimate published in the *New York Times*. I suspect that is an underestimate. Fortunately for the City of New York, most of this cost was borne by FEMA. As far as I'm concerned, the expense of the identification process was well worth it—and I know that it was certainly worth it for the individual families. There are countries where the superhuman effort involved in recovering, collecting, and identifying the remains of thousands of victims would never have happened. Had the WTC attacks taken place even in some advanced nations, it's likely that a few easy identifications would have been made and the remainder of the victims' families would have received nothing, not even the scant comfort of knowing that everything possible had been done to identify their loved one. The site would have been paved over and covered quickly with new buildings, with no regard given to its sanctity.

As the eighteenth-century British statesman William Gladstone eloquently put it, "Show me the manner in which a nation cares for its dead, and I will measure with mathematical exactness, the tender mercies of its people, their loyalty to high ideals, and their regard for the laws of the land." I am very proud that I live in a country that is compassionate enough to have gone above and beyond the norm to identify and return the remains of the WTC victims to their families. If this country is being judged by the way in which it reacted to the WTC attacks, then let the judgers also take note of how we cared for the victims' families. It should be remembered that these were not only American families—they came from a host of countries, and without exception, the families were treated with dignity and respect, and their deceased members received our full attention.

The WTC identification effort was well worth its staggering cost for a second reason. The paths we blazed in using and creating new techniques for victim identification, including the development of new DNA science, have changed the way governments around the world respond to mass fatalities. To some extent, they *had to* change, because by going to extremes in New York City to identify each tiny piece of human tissue, we opened a Pandora's Box: in the wake of each new disaster, victims' families now demand that more be done to locate and identify their loved ones. Some of the techniques we developed have since been used in identifying victims of the tsunami of December 2004. Here in the United States, the procedures we established for the WTC work are being adopted as standard operating procedure for mass-fatality incidents.

Unfortunately they have not yet been fully adopted, a fact I learned when I received calls from friends working to identify the dead in the Hurricane Katrina disaster. Many of the callers had rotated through New York's OCME and worked alongside me during the WTC efforts. Each one mentioned that the Katrina identification effort was being mishandled, that lessons we had learned the hard way during WTC were being ignored. The authorities responsible for the Katrina identification process were evidently reinventing the wheel, which resulted in numerous instances of bungled identifications, of families not being notified in a timely fashion, and of remains being mishandled; many such instances were reported in the press.

It is unfortunate that this great nation of ours, willing to spend huge amounts of money *responding* to a mass-fatality event, won't spend more then a pittance on properly *preparing* for such an event. Perhaps it is the very enormity of such events that prevents us from adequately preparing for them; perhaps it's just a lack of political will. After all, what savvy politician wants to stand up in front of constituents and say, "Yes, it's not a matter of if, but *when* we're going to get hit; and when we do, there will be thousands of fatalities. So we'd better start preparing for that." No one has the courage to take such a stand, because conceding the possibility of another mass disaster would mean admitting that any prevention efforts already underway may well prove to be failures. For instance, in 2004 OCME applied for a grant from the federal government for money to beef up our agency's disaster response capabilities. They turned us down flat with one sentence: "We don't pay for autopsy tables." The federal government might like to believe this, but it's not actually true: when we were cleaning up after 9/11, the federal government did pay for "autopsy tables," and for the work associated with them, to the tune of close to a hundred million dollars.

As I've pointed out, eventually all therapy fails; sooner or later, from whatever cause, every patient dies. Similarly, this country will eventually have another event in which all prevention efforts fail and there are mass fatalities. Whether it comes in the form of a natural disaster like Katrina, or a terrorist act like 9/11, we will get hit again; and next time tens of thousands, or even hundreds of thousands, could die.

We must prepare along two parallel paths: Do everything in our power to prevent such an event, while simultaneously preparing to deal with the inevitable.

Although the stories of heroism and sacrifice will always remain with me, the months that followed 9/11 were also marked by a few scattered instances of cynical and appalling exploitation.

During the time I spent working on the WTC identifications, I testified in two fraud cases prosecuted by the Special Fraud Unit of the Manhattan DA's Office. In the first, a retired FDNY fireman was accused of taking home souvenirs from Ground Zero. The theft was discovered in an unusual way: The man in question lived upstate, and when he put his house up for sale, an off-duty New York state trooper went to see it as a potential buyer. When he stepped into the firefighter's living room, he was shocked to see a large blown-up picture of the retired firefighter holding up a piece of human remains at Ground Zero as though it were a hunting trophy. Clearly oblivious to the cop's disgust, the firefighter went on to brag about his important role in the recovery effort—including how he had taken many other items away from the site. The trooper reported the incident to his commanding officers, and shortly thereafter investigators posing as a young couple looking for a home entered the firefighter's residence and found other souvenirs from Ground Zero—a piece of a radio, a credit card, and more. After the state police arrested him, they transferred the case to New York City, where the theft had occurred.

Before the trial, the assistant DA showed me the stolen items and the large photo, complete with a date-stamp. The remains were so clearly visible in the picture that we decided to determine if we could locate them, and if they had ever been identified. Using an extremely detailed description produced from the photo by anthropologist Amy Mundorff, we searched the database for any remains matching that description that had been brought in to OCME between ten days before the date on the photo and twenty days after the date. There were no matches. In desperation, we hand-checked each remain that arrived during those thirty days, but still there was no sign of the remains so clearly seen in his hands in that photo. The remains had evidently never been brought in to OCME. Now we had another concern. Had this man actually stolen the remains as a macabre souvenir of his brief stint at the site? If he didn't, where was the body part?

On the witness stand, I laid out for the court how identifications were made, and gave my expert-witness opinion that the fireman's behavior constituted more than theft, because it could have interfered with the making of identifications. (There was no way to say positively that it had interfered with any specific identification.) For technical reasons related to the type of crime the man was charged with, my testimony was not allowed into evidence; in the end, he was convicted of petty theft, but not of obstruction of justice, which I felt would have been a far more just decision. To me, this case was an awful example of the necessity of leaving crimes scenes pristine and untrammeled. The convicted thief was questioned repeatedly, but he always denied taking the remains seen in the photo. I would like to believe him, but will always wonder what happened to those particular remains.

In the second case, the same fraud unit prosecuted a man from Nigeria who had invented a dead wife who supposedly had died in the WTC. Her remains had not been identified, and the documents he had brought to the Family Assistance Center were in bad shape; the church back home had burned down, he said, and all he could obtain were copies of copies. Before his fraud was exposed, he did obtain some money from the Red Cross, but he was stopped before he got his hands on the larger pot of money for the families of victims.

This and other such cases raised my indignation, because I knew how much the real families of the WTC dead needed the money that was being amassed to assist them. Yet the defrauders were penny ante, small-time criminals compared to what is alleged to have happened right in my own office. In the summer of 2005, two longtime employees of OCME—the director of Management Information System and his girlfriend, the director of our medical records unit—were arrested and charged with stealing *millions* of dollars earmarked for the development of WTC computer systems, specifically for DNA matching software. When Bob Shaler, the director of the DNA lab, learned of this, he told the New York *Daily News* that the theft *must* have interfered with the WTC identification effort. He was in a position to know that, but I must report that the official position of New York City and OCME was that the alleged theft and the loss of millions of dollars in no way impeded the WTC identification effort. All I can say is that while the missing funds did not directly impact my work in the Incident Command Center, I'm inclined to share Shaler's view. Looking back, the alleged theft may explain why some DNA identifications took so long to make, or were never made—the computer systems simply were never developed.

Ultimately, even if this theft is proven to have occurred as alleged, and further proven to have impacted the identification effort, I believe that it will only have been a delay rather then an irrevocable stoppage. The OCME is committed never to cease its efforts to identify the remains of 9/11 victims. And if OCME keeps at the identification effort as promised, sooner or later every possible identification will be made. It's just a matter of technology and time.

Around eighteen months after the disaster, in early 2003, the crew working on the WTC identifications was sharply reduced. It had become more difficult for the agency to obtain funds for the task from New York's City Hall, and OCME had its regular work to deal with; death had not taken a holiday. Dr. Hirsch decided it was time to start returning OCME to normalcy. The first step was to reclaim the agency's conference room that I was still using as the Incident Command Center. A diminished Incident Command Center staff of about fifteen, including Katie Sullivan and other stalwarts, was moved out of the conference room and into a doublewide trailer parked on Thirtieth Street alongside the OCME headquarters. Some additional staff members like Amy Mundorff returned to regular work but spent at least half their time on WTC-related work, while about twenty additional people continued to toil on WTC matters in the OCME DNA lab.

There was still plenty of WTC identification work. New identifications were still being made, though considerably fewer of them, and because these identifications were more difficult to confirm, they required more intense scrutiny and administrative review before the families could be notified. Also, secondary or additional remains identifications were constantly coming in, and families had to be notified of them.

And there was another complication: for many of the families, life was moving on. Once I notified a widow that we had finally identified her husband, only to learn that she had already remarried. I remember feeling somewhat shocked, until I realized that it was almost two years after the event. Why shouldn't a young person have moved on and re-married? Still, such second marriages required a shift in our approach: henceforth, in talking to such widows and widowers, we used a look-before-you-leap conversational strategy.

We made a point of raising such issues at our regular meetings with the family groups. We reported to them on our progress and used them as a sounding board for ideas on how to handle such sensitive situations. Interestingly, some families kept coming to our regular meetings after their own loved ones had been identified, although most of those who had received an identification eventually drifted away. Those who remained offered increasingly sophisticated questions about, say, the efficacy of mitochondrial matches, or the number of loci necessary to make us feel certain enough of a match to issue an identification.

"So what are you doing still to find my loved one?" a family member would ask at an individual session. I'd sometimes use little yellow sticky notes to demonstrate by analogy how we were working with composite DNA methods. Covering a portrait of the deceased with a dozen or more of the sticky notes—enough to obscure the face of the person in the photo—I'd tell a family that a mitochondrial match might allow us to remove three of the dozen sticky notes, revealing some of the face; another technique would allow us to remove another two sticky notes; and so on, until enough of the portrait had been un-covered so that the face was recognizable and identifiable.

While working with the families, I took part in the making of two documentary films about 9/11 and its aftermath. One was put together by the organization of families from Cantor Fitzgerald, the firm that had suffered the greatest personnel loss in the disaster. Danielle Gardner, who had lost a brother in the disaster, was the principal in making that documentary about the event and the work of identifying the victims. In this effort, she was supported by Edie Lutnick and Howard Lutnick, who had also lost their brother. Howard, the CEO of Cantor Fitzgerald, behaved in an exemplary way; he and Edie formed Cantor Relief, an organization (which he funds) dedicated to helping his company's families cope and recover as best they can from the tragedy. No company did more for its employees than Cantor Fitzgerald.

A second documentary was spurred into being by a chance encounter. Several months after the disaster, filmmaker Marc Levin was riding in a New York City taxi when its driver, a man from a Middle Eastern, predominantly Muslim country, began pontificating that the WTC disaster was the result of a Jewish conspiracy, a plot undertaken by American and Israeli Jews, and that the proof of the conspiracy was that no Jews had died in the bombings. According to this ridiculous notion, all the Jews in the WTC had been notified the night before not to go to work on the day the planes were to hit the towers. Levin began arguing with the cab driver and asked him where he had gotten his information. The cab driver waved a copy of *The Protocols of the Elders of Zion,* saying, "The proof is all in here!" After obtaining a copy of the legendary anti-Semitic tract for himself, Levin was flummoxed that such nonsense was still being actively published and, even more mind-boggling, was being taken seriously by millions of people around the world. Incensed by the book's allegations, Marc decided to make a documentary about the *Protocols,* the resurgence of anti-Semitism after 9/11, and the true identity of the victims of the WTC bombings.

For the documentary, I was able to state authoritatively on camera that hundreds of Jews died in the attacks on the WTC. From the list of the missing and identified dead, and conversations with the families, I estimated that easily 20 percent of the victims of the bombings had been Jewish. My count was not official, since OCME emphatically did not collect or maintain records of victims' religions. Even had we done so, there would have been some difficulty in figuring out who was a Jew and who was not. But I had my own, very simple criterion: if Hitler would have considered a particular person a Jew, and on that basis would have sent this person to their death, they were Jewish enough for me. (Indeed, there is anecdotal evidence that the buildings may have been chosen because the Muslim terrorists wanted to target a heavily Jewish industry.) Having had hundreds of conversations with family members, I amassed ample anecdotal evidence to back this claim, and I still have my list of "probably Jewish" names on file in case anyone wants to challenge my conclusion.

Although many Americans seem to have overlooked the fact, a relatively high number of British citizens perished in the WTC attacks. One result of this unhappy circumstance was that I had frequent contact with Patrick Owens, Her Majesty's Counsel at the British Consulate in New York. In 2004 I suggested to him that Great Britain recognize and acknowledge the terrific work done by our British computer expert, Adrian Jones, in this disaster. To Adrian's delight, and mine, at Christmas 2004 he was knighted and awarded the title of Member of the Order of the British Empire by Queen Elizabeth II.

Adrian's commendation came as I was nearing a turning point of my own. Early in 2005, I formally left the post of director of WTC operations and returned to my regular work at OCME. I was content to do so in part because I knew that my successor, Katie Sullivan, would do a superb job.

On the first Sunday in April 2005, at the church of St. Francis of Assisi in mid-Manhattan, a memorial service and appreciation ceremony was held by many of the families of the victims of the WTC terrorist attacks to honor the work of the New York City ME's Office. It was a kind of unofficial end to the long identification process; we had exhausted virtually every avenue for identifying the remains, and it was clear to everyone, including the families, that no further new identifications would be made. A formal OCME letter to that effect would be mailed a few months later to all the WTC families, stating that while we maintained our commitment to never stop trying to identify the victims of 9/11, we had reached the limits of current science. We pledged to the families that we would resume the identification effort when new technologies made it feasible.

The event in April was set into motion with a single e-mail from Bill Doyle, leader of a WTC family group in Staten Island, to the leadership of all the other family groups, who in turn sent out e-mails to their memberships. As a result of these communications, representatives from hundreds of WTC families showed up at the church to hear a few speakers. I was privileged to be one of those scheduled to address the crowd. It was an occasion I wouldn't have missed for the world, an acknowledgement of the most difficult, most arduous, and most rewarding work that I have ever done—and, I suspected, that I would ever do.

When I stood up on the dais and moved to the rostrum, I grabbed Katie Sullivan and pulled her along with me. The members of the families stood up too, giving us a standing ovation. It was one of the most moving moments of my life.

While in principle I was returning to regular work at OCME, in an important sense I was unable to return to the world I had left behind. While I had been concentrating on the WTC effort, the position of director of identifications and communications for OCME had been filled by another. Moreover, I had grown beyond that level of management during my time running the 9/11 effort.

Yet it was now equally clear that I was not going to achieve my earlier goal of becoming director of medicolegal investigations. I had been on that track before WTC and, at the time, I could think of no greater career aspiration. During my three and a half years of intensive work on the WTC effort, however, the old director had retired and was replaced by a contemporary of mine, and by the time I emerged from my tunnel, she had been in place for two years. It was obvious that she was going to remain in that job for quite a while. At this time, it was also made clear to me by senior members of OCME's administration that they intended to take the agency beyond the WTC identification efforts. "I hate WTC," one muttered to me, "I hate the families."

Though I was shocked at the harshness of this statement, I actually understood where it came from. The OCME had become too exclusively focused on the WTC dead, and on servicing their families, and now it would finally have to return to the more broad-based role it was designed to fill. Our work with the WTC families had involved procedures that went far beyond the accustomed role of an ME's office. It was special work with special demands, requiring continual contact for months and years until every identification issue was addressed. But that was a very different assignment from the work we had trained to do, and it was time for the office to turn back to its traditional model.

Since no suitable management position for me existed within the hierarchy of the agency, one was created: director of special projects. Now, in Clive Cussler's bestselling books, the "director of special projects" in his fictional government maritime agency NUMA has an awful lot to do, and every moment of it is exciting. Not so with the director of special projects for OCME. I was put in charge of the development of a software program that would integrate every function and every department of OCME. It was diverting, but it simply never felt like the most rewarding work I could be doing.

I did my job, but I grew restless. At length, I found it increasingly difficult to be at OCME after the WTC effort was over. That had been the defining investigation of my forensic career, and anything else I could envision myself doing at OCME paled by comparison. The echoes of the WTC effort rang in my ears and followed me everywhere I went in the hallways of the building.

One evening at home, I received a call from a WTC family member, wondering why she couldn't get beyond her grief. It was the birthday of the brother she had lost in the bombings. For both of us, 9/11 had become so ingrained in our collective consciousness that we couldn't help but see continual reminders of it everywhere. It sometimes seemed impossible to have even a brief conversation without bringing up 9/11 in some way, and a thousand times a day there were references to it in every type of media. Random searches at the airports, and then on the New York subways, were taxing reminders of our shared vulnerability. The collective need to touch the touchstone, to bring up the pain on every possible occasion, and to connect it to every possible subject, was the reason that 9/11 could not fade from this woman's consciousness. After that phone call I realized consciously, for the first time, what my subconscious had been trying to tell me for months—the same was true for me. It was unhealthy for me to remain at OCME. Like the families, I too had to get past 9/11.

I wasn't alone. Katie Sullivan decided to leave OCME in the early summer of 2005, returning with her husband to Virginia, where they had both grown up. Katie also went back to teaching and opened an organic foods kitchen.

Amy Mundorff also left to complete her doctoral studies at the University of British Columbia on a Trudeau Scholarship. She had long felt that others in her profession looked askance at anyone who lacked a doctorate and a university affiliation, and despite her extraordinary work surveying twenty thousand pieces of human remains in the WTC effort, she knew she needed the ultimate sheepskin to prove her forensic expertise to some academics.

Bob Shaler retired from OCME to become the head of a new program at Penn State University that trains crime scene investigators, an innovative program that will likely make Penn State the center of forensic education for the northeast.

Mark Flomenbaum also left, and accepted the position of CME for the state of Massachusetts. Tom Brondolo, the deputy commissioner who had headed up our WTC computer effort, resigned from OCME and is now in private practice as a consultant.

I knew that all of these good people, too, needed to move on; the WTC identification effort had been the culmination of their best work at OCME, a pinnacle that would never again be reached. Still, I could never quite shake the sense that they and WTC had been collectively nudged out the OCME door. I, too, was feeling the nudge. By summer of 2005, of the half-dozen people who had led the WTC identification effort, only I remained. I had just turned forty, and I was whiling away my time in a job that would never command my passion.

It was at that moment that OCME's director of information management and director of records was arrested in an astonishing embezzlement case. The alleged criminal activity had evidently begun long before 9/11, but had heated up considerably thereafter. This totally unexpected event—unexpected, at least, by me—all but sidelined OCME's effort to develop the all-encompassing software program for the agency that I was directing.

I continued on at OCME for a few more months, but soon it was painfully obvious that I was spinning my wheels. Wasting time is something I'm not very good at. I'm a good manager, but I never liked being a bureaucrat. I needed a new direction. And so at last I decided to resign from OCME at the end of 2005, to pursue other projects, including this book.

I never held a more exciting job than medicolegal investigator. I went to work every morning with a sense of keen anticipation, looking forward to solving whatever complex challenges the world would throw at me that day. And when finally the challenge became helping the ME's office respond to the tragedy at the WTC, the opportunity to apply my skill and experience and help people every day—to make order out of chaos—was to me, little short of perfect.

ACKNOWLEDGMENTS

I WISH TO thank a wonderful group of current and former employees of the office of Chief Medical Examiner, City of New York, who encouraged me to write this book: Amy Mundorff, Harry Hahn, Kenny Dotson, Esther Arrington, Tammie Natali, and Jimmy Meyer, and a most special thanks to my dear friend Dr. Robert Shaler for sharing his recollections and standing with me during the rough times during and after September 11th.

Thanks to FDNY's Chief of Dept. Sal Cassano, Chief Fire Marshal Louie Garcia, and to NYPD's Sgt. Joe Blozis, Detectives Hal Sherman and James Nucifioro, and to Deputy Commissioner Bradford Billet of the Mayor's Office, for helping me with fact checking and for their support.

I also would like to thank Mel Berger, literary agent at the William Morris Agency, for showing me the path, and gently pushing me along it.

I am deeply indebted to the members of my Brotherhood Synagogue family, for their love and support along the way, most especially to Dan Alder and Phil Rothman. A heartfelt thanks to Roz Weinman, former executive producer of *Law & Order* for opening more doors than I can count.

And lastly many thanks to Cal Morgan, Matt Harper, and the crew of the Regan imprint at HarperCollins for their splendid work, at some odd hours of the night.

SHIYA RIBOWSKY

INDEX